NURSE PRACTITIONER PROTOCOLS

SECOND EDITION

By Matthew M. Cohen, M.D., FAFP
and
Anni Lanigan, ARNP, FNP-C

SUNBELT
MEDICAL
PUBLISHERS

NOTICE: The authors and publisher of this book have, as far as it is possible to do so, taken care to make certain that recommendations regarding the evaluation and treatment of patients and the use of drugs are correct and compatible with the standard practice of medicine at the time of publication. However, knowledge in medical science is constantly changing. As new information becomes available, changes in evaluation, treatment, and the use of drugs become necessary and protocols should be revised accordingly. The authors and publisher disavow any responsibility for failure to diagnose or for the outcomes of patients to whom these protocols are applied.

ISBN 0-924381-07-8

SUNBELT MEDICAL PUBLISHERS
P.O. Box 13512
Tallahassee, FL 32317-3512

DEDICATION

To the spirited nurses who pioneered the expansion of the nurse practitioner role, and to those doctors who have supported them along the way.

TABLE OF CONTENTS

TABLE OF CONTENTS (CONTINUED)

TABLE OF CONTENTS (CONTINUED)

TABLE OF CONTENTS (CONTINUED)

TABLE OF CONTENTS (CONTINUED)

PREFACE

When we wrote our first edition of <u>Nurse Practitioner Protocols</u> in 1989 we were unclear how well it would be received and just who would buy it. Since the writing of our second edition is being prompted by the sell-out of the original edition, at the least we have been encouraged that there is a need for this type of book.

We've sent books to nearly every state in the U.S. and to as many rural locations as urban ones. We have shipped orders overseas. We've been grateful to have the book selected as a text or for text material for several dozen nurse practitioner training programs.

This response has been exciting and illuminating. It confirms what we already know--that nurse practitioners are playing an active and major role in the provision of health care in this country. They are doing this in myriad ways and in settings as diverse as the population itself is.

This book, which is a collaborative effort, reflects the relationship of trust, teamwork, and interdependence that we have in our practice. As we have grown from one family physician and one family family nurse practitioner to one family physician and three family nurse practitioners, we have realized the value of using <u>Nurse Practitioner Protocols</u> as a tool to focus our communications to establish an integrated and updated clinical approach to the care of our patients.

The management protocols have grown to include more preventive care and wellness guidelines and we've added some additional diagnoses that we believe still reflect the most common problems seen in a family practice setting.

This book will hopefully be used as a workbook which you will feel free to write in, update, or amend. The blank lines in the therapeutic section are meant to encourage the establishment of an individual formulary for your practice. As with the last edition, an important goal of <u>Nurse Practitioner Protocols</u> is to facilitate communication between nurse practitioners and their physician supervisors or consultants. Additionally, it can serve as criteria to establish acceptable standards of care for peer review or for evaluation of your solo practice.

We have left the format the same in this second edition as it has served well to organize the protocols and be amenable to the tailoring process where you adapt the protocol to fit your practice needs.

Again, we emphasize that this is not a comprehensive text for the nurse practitioner. Its focus is on common problems seen in primary care settings, particularly as seen by the authors. The authors were assisted in identifying the problems included by various references.[1] [2] [3] There should be an initial and ongoing process in each type of practice in which the nurse practitioner and the physician consultant or supervisor assure each other that the problems seen and the treatment given are within the range of the nurse practitioner's knowledge and skills. There should be on-premise access to and familiarity with current editions of standard references applicable to your practice.

There will always be a diversity and complexity to the care of human beings that precludes using a stringent "cookbook" type approach. We hope this book is interpreted as a flexible and usable guide rather than a hindrance to the use of good judgment and independent practice style.

Matthew M. Cohen, M.D., F.A.F.P.
Anni Lanigan, A.R.N.P., F.N.P.-C.

---

[1]International Classification of Disease. Revision 9, Clinical Modification (ICD-9-CM). Ann Arbor, MI: Commission on Professional and Hospital Activities, 1978.

[2]National Center for Health Statistics. The National Ambulatory Medical Care Survey, 1977 Summary. Hyattsville, MD: Public Health Service, April 23, 1980.

[3]Schneeweiss, R., Rosenblatt, R., Cherkin, D., et al. Diagnostic Clusters: A New Tool for Analyzing the Content of Ambulatory Medical Care. Med. Care, 1983; 21:105.

INTRODUCTION

This collection of protocols was designed to be useful for nurse practitioners in organizing their therapeutic interactions, communicating with physician consultants, and serving as a reference that is easily accessible. The authors have purposefully designed the format of <u>Nurse Practitioner Protocols</u> to allow tailoring to your practice needs and to your training and orientation.

Each subject is organized into an evaluative section and a therapeutic section, integrated in a problem-oriented fashion. We feel that the problem-oriented approach is a standard that serves well to focus practitioners in all types of settings across the country.

By intent, the authors have not written a comprehensive textbook. Consequently the protocols are succinctly designed to direct and cue the nurse practitioner toward both signs and symptoms and the critical analysis of this information while setting guidelines for health education, therapeutic measures, pharmacotherapy, physician consultation, or referrals. Since the protocols use the S.O.A.P. structure, they should help you to organize the progress notes going into the patient's chart.

When we originally chose an open-ended format we intended to create a device that would instigate focused interaction and communication between the nurse practitioner and the consulting/supervising physician. Since then it has become clear that many nurse practitioners have solo practices, partnerships, or other independent practice arrangements. We continue to believe there is a need for such a tool, both for those who work in large institutions or practices where they are supervised and those who are practicing independently. For those in solo or nurse practitioner owned practices it can be a guide to help you analyze your standards of care, audit yourself or provide research data.

Optimally, this book should be reviewed together and filled in by the nurse practitioner(s) and the physician(s) that they consult with. If you go through this process we can assure you that questions will arise, differences in opinion will surface, and some new insights will be gained by all.

Try to take the time to do this. Be flexible, feel free to use this as a workbook. Fill in the spaces, jot reminders or "pearls" in the margins, update with new therapies, referrals, etc. Please see the actual examples from our collaborative practice from the previous edition on the following pages.

The (MIS) abbreviation following the pharmacological agent spaces is to remind you to give medical information sheets as well as verbal instructions when prescribing or dispensing. The heading **Referral** is most often followed by space for you to address your practice circumstance for that problem. There are exceptions where the authors felt strongly that established standards of care must be met.

For a family practice, we feel that most common diagnoses have been included. For other practices, you may want to pull those subjects not appropriate to your practice or additional protocols. A formatted page is available for you to photocopy and use to organize other subjects into this protocol notebook before your practice.

The protocols begin with a newly expanded preventive care section. Obviously the frequency of visits and preventive health measures will vary with a patient's individual or family needs and risk factors.

The chapter on emergencies was included to be certain that you and your staff have taken the time to plan for, in particular, a life-threatening emergency, should it occur on the premises.

The last section has some patient instruction sheets that can be easily reproduced and given to your patients. We believe that written instructions are invaluable. Add your own, as we are a long way from being able to offer one with each protocol.

Any attempt to establish standard protocols for common problems is limited by the fact that problems vary according to population, geography, climate, and other factors. Even the use of the word "protocol" is subject to debate about its meaning, ambiguity, or political ramifications. Nevertheless, we sincerely hope that <u>Nurse Practitioner Protocols</u> will be helpful to you. We desire feedback and suggestions. If future editions incorporate your suggestions, you will be duly acknowledged.

Asthma, Adults

EVALUATION/DIAGNOSTIC PROTOCOL
Subjective
History. General and respiratory history. Emphasis on history of allergic disorders, both personal and familial. Try to ascertain precipitating factor (infection the most common, but also consider allergy, environmental change, exercise). It is important to assess family history of allergic disorders. Remember that more than 10% of asthmatics may never wheeze but instead have a history of coughing and have been labeled as having recurring acute bronchitis. Obtain meticulous history of medications used in the past 36 hours, including amounts and times taken.

Objective
Physical Examination. General appearance, vital signs, ENT, chest.

Lab. Laboratory tests may not be necessary. For infection, consider chest X-ray and CBC. To assess function, consider pulmonary function studies/simple spirometry. Consider theophylline level.

Assess severity, therapeutic needs and asthma education needs. **Differential Diagnosis:** LTB, bronchitis, pneumonia. **Complications:** Pulmonary infection, hypoxia, respiratory failure, pneumothorax.

PLAN/MANAGEMENT PROTOCOL
General Measures. Explain the nature of asthma to patient and give reinforcing educational literature. Emphasize the need to avoid exposure to all inhalants and tobacco smoke in particular. Advise allergy proofing (see Allergy Proofing). Ultimately, for the adult with persistent symptoms establish both maintenance and contingency plans. Carefully construct criteria for use of the latter.

Specific Measures. ACUTE MEASURES (Physician Consultation)
or Susphrine mls ALC
If pulse less than 120, consider subcut. injection(s) of _Epinephrine 1:1000, 3m/SQ_. (Check P and BP, before and 10 minutes after). (Caution patient about immediate effects of this injection), or a nebulizer inhalation of _____N/A_____.

Consider injection of corticosteroid _Decadron 4-8 mg IM_ *(MIS).

Consider oral antibiotic Rx _see acute Bronchitis choices pg 5-5_ *(MIS).

MAINTENANCE THERAPY
Choose from oral theophylline Rx and/or Rx for inhaled or oral beta adrenergic stimulator _TheoDur 200-450mg Q12h ; Proventil Repetabs 4mg Q12h. or inhaler_ *(MIS)
(Albuteral) _Proventil Inhaler ii puffs Q4h._ and/or
Rx for cromolyn _Intal Inhaler ii puffs QID or TID_ *(MIS)
or oral or inhaled corticosteroid _Beclomethasone Inhaler ii puffs TID_ *(MIS).

    Do not use sedative tranquilizers, cough suppressants, or antihistamines without physician consultation.

Physician Consultation. On all newly diagnosed or difficult to manage asthmatics.

Referral. Upon advice of physician to allergist or pulmonary internist.

Immediate Transfer. For severe respiratory distress. Nurse practitioner and physician must define criteria (e.g. pulse above 140 or ____) to _TCH or TMRMC_.

Follow-up Plan. After the acute illness in _1-5_ day(s) and when on *beginning* maintenance regime every _2_ week(s)/month(s). Monitor serum drug levels as indicated. **Caution patients ask for help if worsening on maintenance therapy and not helped by contingency plan.**

* unless allergic, contraindicated, or pregnant/lactating	_LH 1/21/91_ Physician ARNP _mK J-JP-90_	Initials _MM_ _ALC_	Date _3/16/89_ _3/16/89_

Contact Dermatitis

EVALUATION/DIAGNOSTIC PROTOCOL

Subjective

History. Symptoms, course (initial appearance, ascertain possible exposure to irritant or allergen as well as aggravating and alleviating factors).

Objective

Physical Examination. Thorough skin examination note location and distribution of (in order of severity from minimum to maximum) erythema, vesicles, blisters, erosions, ulcers. Patches and streaks are the sine qua non.

Lab. Usually not necessary, though consideration should be given to herpes culture.

Assess severity and possible etiology. **Differential Diagnosis:** Atopic, seborrheic, and other vesicular/bullous dermatoses, dermatophyte infections and scabies. **Complications:** Excoriations and secondary infections.

PLAN/MANAGEMENT PROTOCOL

General Measures. Remove the irritant. In the future avoid the contact allergen (remind patient that even with treatment it may be several weeks before resolution appears. Use only mild soaps when washing.

Cold compressing _Aveeno oatmeal colloidal solution; Burows solution_

Soothing creams and lotions _Calamine lotion._

Specific Measures.

Consider oral antihistamine OTC and Rx _Benadryl 25-50 mg n dose for wgt & age_ *(MIS).
Atarax or Vistaril — dose for wgt & age

Consider corticosteroid, topical OTC or Rx _Cl II III IV V or VI usually II_ *(MIS). Be certain to limit use and potency on young children and on any face or other area likely to be damaged permanently.

or

Short course oral Rx _Prednisone 2 mg/kg/day   n Decadron .5 mg/kg/day q 8 hr_ *(MIS).

Physician Consultation. For severe cases, therapeutic complications, therapeutic failure or diagnostic doubt.

Adults: Prednisone 10-40 mg per dose BID OR TID ē meals   OR

Referral. Dermatologist for therapeutic failure. _Depo-Medrol 40-80 mg DEEP IM_
Decadron 4-8 mg IM initially, then begin oral ↑

Immediate Transfer. May be necessary for caustic contactants.

Follow-up Plan. _1-5_ days if no improvement, sooner if worse.

* unless allergic, contraindicated or pregnant/lactating

	Physician ARNP	Initials	Date
	2-22-90	MC	6/8/89
	EA 1/11/91	ALC	6/8/89

Title

EVALUATION/DIAGNOSTIC PROTOCOL
Subjective
History.

Objective
Physical Examination.

Lab.

Assessment/Differential Diagnosis/Complications

PLAN/MANAGEMENT PROTOCOL
General Measures.

Specific Measures.

Physician Consultation.

Referral.

Immediate Transfer.

Follow-up Plan.

ACKNOWLEDGMENTS

This collaborative work is an outgrowth of a collaborative practice of Family Medicine. We would like to thank those who work or have worked with us in this practice and who have been so supportive of this project: Janet Lindeman, Judy Kleynen, Peggy West, Mary Anne Ernst, Debbie Vasquez, Susan Gaines, Linda Brown, Pam Abbott, and Tracy Wright.

Our colleagues have helped with advice, encouragement, and some have even painstakingly read drafts of the work in progress: T. E. Enoch, M.D.; M. E. Shamis, M.D.; W. P. Kaufman, M.D.; M. Kung, A.R.N.P.; E. Heuler, A.R.N.P.

Practicing medicine in a community is a collaborative effort. Accordingly, several other colleagues served as contributors: D. Hansen, M.D., P. Catinella, M.D., K. Skilling, A.R.N.P., and V. Spitzer, A.R.N.P.

Two people were directly involved in the preparation of this project: Juliana Klein, who helped with preparation of manuscripts and redrafting; and especially Kathy Watkins, projects manager, who supervised every aspect of production of this project.

Most important, our families continue to encourage our endeavors. Without their support and patience, <u>Nurse Practitioner Protocols</u> could not have been completed. Thank you, Leslie, Jessie, Gabe, Van, Ian, and Noah.

CHAPTER 1
PREVENTIVE HEALTH CARE

Preventive Health Care, Children

● = After recommendations A.A.P. in the standard manner or method.
e = Electively employed by authors.
s = Subjectively determined by history.

[1] American Academy of Pediatrics Guidelines for Health Supervision.
[2] Sex Education and Information Council of the United States.

The chart plots preventive health care activities against age, grouped into WEEKS (2, 4, 8, 12, 16, 20, 24), MONTHS (7, 8, 9, 10, 11, 12, 15, 18, 21, 24, 27, 30, 33, 36), and YEARS (4, 5, 6, 7, 8, 9, 10, 11, 12, 13, 14, 15, 16, 17, 18, 19, 20).

Row categories:

SUBJECTIVE
- Update Hx

OBJECTIVE
- Complete PEx
- Ht, Wt, (HC until 12 months)
- BP, P
- Visual Scr.
- Hearing Scr.
- Developmental Scr.
- Behavioral Scr.

LAB
- Hered./Metabolic Scr.
- Hct
- U/A
- Tb Test

ANTICIPATORY GUIDANCE [1]
- Feeding/Dietary
- Growth & Development
- Behavior
- Safety
- Sex Education [2]

THERAPY
- Immunizations

Preventive Health Care, Children

WEEKS | MONTHS | YEARS

WEEKS: 2 4 8 12 16 20 24

MONTHS: 7 8 9 10 11 12 15 18 21 24 27 30 33 36

YEARS: 4 5 6 7 8 9 10 11 12 13 14 15 16 17 18 19 20

SUBJECTIVE
Update Hx

OBJECTIVE
Complete PEx
Ht, Wt, (HC until 12 months)
BP, P
Visual Scr.
Hearing Scr.
Developmental Scr.
Behavioral Scr.

LAB
Hered./Metabolic Scr.
Hct
U/A
Tb Test

ANTICIPATORY GUIDANCE [1]
Feeding/Dietary
Growth & Development
Behavior
Safety
Sex Education [2]

THERAPY
Immunizations

CHILD HEALTH SUPERVISION
2 TO 4 WEEKS

The authors have included for distribution immediately after birth instructions sheets entitled <u>Your Newborn</u> and <u>Newborn Care</u> in Chapter 16: Patient Instructions.

EVALUATION/DIAGNOSTIC PROTOCOL
Subjective
Interval History. Which parents or significant others have accompanied the child? How is the baby described? How is the baby sleeping? Has there been any illness? Have there been any accidents?

General Nutritional. How is the baby nursing? Is he/she on formula? How much and how often? Are there any feeding difficulties? Describe elimination pattern. Vitamins? Fluoride? (Support programs WIC.)

Interval Key Family Checks. How is Mom's health? Is she able to rest? Is there outside support present? What are her feelings? What are Dad's feelings? What are the siblings' ages and how are they adjusting? Is there tobacco, alcohol, or drug usage in the home? What are the child care plans?

Objective
Physical Examination. Vital signs (T and Wt, Wt%, Ht, Ht%, HC, HC%), general appearance, head (fontanelle), eyes (red reflex), ears (TMs), nose, oropharynx, neck, chest (breasts), lungs, cardiovascular (femoral pulse, S2), abdomen (umbilicus), genitalia, musculoskeletal (hip click/clunk), skin, lymph nodes, neurologic (moro).

Development. Cuddles? Regards face? Head up (prone)? Responds to sound? Equal movements? Follows to midline? Describe parent-child interaction?

Lab. Neonatal screening results or repeat.

<u>Assess</u> the child's status.

<u>Assess</u> the family's status.

PLAN/MANAGEMENT PROTOCOL
General Measures/Anticipatory Guidance. Discuss sleep pattern (reassure parents during the second month that sleep patterns improve and are more predictable), nutritional practices, and elimination patterns. Emphasize cuddling and loving (encourage age appropriate play and stimulation). Give permission for babysitters and parent private time. Discuss crying and infant communication skills.
   Discuss safety measures, including car safety seat and safe practices, crib safety, fire safety, preventing falls.
   Anticipate colic and diaper rash questions. Briefly review fever management and temperature taking. Distribute companion educational materials and reference list.

Specific Measures. Anticipatory immunization education materials.

Physician Consultation. At practitioner's discretion.

Follow-up Plan. _____ weeks.

Taken from <u>Ambulatory Child Health Care Protocols</u> to be published by Sunbelt Medical Publishers in January 1992.

CHILD HEALTH SUPERVISION
2 MONTHS

EVALUATION/DIAGNOSTIC PROTOCOL

Subjective

Interval History. Which parents or significant others have accompanied the child? How is the baby described? How is the baby sleeping? Has there been any illness? Have there been any accidents? Has the baby had colic? How is the baby seeing/hearing?

General Nutritional. How is the baby nursing? Is he/she on formula? How much and how often? Are there any feeding difficulties? Describe elimination pattern. Vitamins? Fluoride? (Support programs WIC.)

Interval Key Family Checks. How is Mom's health? Are she and the infant on a regular schedule? How much is Dad involved? Is there a support system for the family? Are the parents getting out? How is the family adjusting? Has Mom gone back to school or work? What are the child care arrangements?

Objective

Physical Examination. Vital signs (T and Wt, Wt%, Ht, Ht%, HC, HC%), general appearance, head (fontanelle), eyes (red reflex), ears (TMs), nose, oropharynx, neck, chest (breasts), lungs, cardiovascular (femoral pulse, S2), abdomen, genitalia, musculoskeletal (hip click/clunk), skin, lymph nodes, neurologic (moro).

Development. Smiles? Vocalizes? Head up (prone)? Listens to bell? Describe parent-child interaction?

Lab.

Assess the child's status.

Assess the family's status.

PLAN/MANAGEMENT PROTOCOL

General Measures/Anticipatory Guidance. Discuss sleep pattern (anticipate increasing nighttime sleep), nutritional practices (nurse or formula feed solely, solids not necessary), and elimination patterns. Emphasize cuddling and loving (encourage age appropriate play and stimulation). Give permission for babysitters and parent private time.

Discuss safety measures, including car safety seat and safe practices, crib safety, fire safety, pet cautions, preventing falls, walkers. Emphasize that the hot water temperature should be less than 125° F.

Discuss skin care and anticipate rash questions. Distribute companion educational materials and reference list.

Specific Measures. DPT #1, OPV #1, HIB.[1] Immunization education materials and releases.

Physician Consultation. At practitioner's discretion.

Follow-up Plan. _____ months.

---

[1] Consult USPHS schedule as frequency of immunization varies with type of vaccine and age immunization is initiated.

Taken from Ambulatory Child Health Care Protocols to be published by Sunbelt Medical Publishers in January 1992.

CHILD HEALTH SUPERVISION
4 MONTHS

EVALUATION/DIAGNOSTIC PROTOCOL

Subjective

Interval History. Which parents or significant others have accompanied the child? How is the baby described? How is the baby sleeping? Has there been illness? Accidents? Are the eyes always straight? Has the baby started reaching out? Has there been any reaction to immunizations?

General Nutritional. How is the baby nursing? Is he/she on formula? How much and how often? Has the baby started on solids? Are there any feeding difficulties? Describe elimination pattern. Vitamins? Fluoride? (Support programs WIC.)

Interval Key Family Checks. How is Mom's health? Are she and the infant on a regular schedule? Are the siblings adjusting? Has Mom gone back to school or work? What is the child care arrangement? Is there a support system? Is Dad involved?

Objective

Physical Examination. Vital signs (T and Wt, Wt%, Ht, Ht%, HC, HC%), general appearance, head (fontanelle), eyes (red reflex), visual tracking, ears (TMs), nose, oropharynx, neck, chest (breasts), lungs, cardiovascular (femoral pulse), abdomen, genitalia, musculoskeletal (hip click/clunk), skin, lymph nodes, neurologic.

Development. Squeals? Grasps? Rolls over? Head erect on sitting? Follows 180 degrees? Hands together? Parent-child interaction?

Lab.

Assess the child's status.

Assess the family's status.

PLAN/MANAGEMENT PROTOCOL

General Measures/Anticipatory Guidance. Discuss nutrition. Discuss safety: car, falls, tub, houseproofing. Discuss play patterns, sleep patterns. Discuss colds. Discuss day care. Emphasize the need for a fire escape plan. Distribute companion education and reference list.

Specific Measures. DPT #2, OPV #2, HIB.[1] Immunization education materials and releases.

Physician Consultation. At practitioner's discretion.

Follow-up Plan. _____ months.

---

[1]Consult USPHS schedule as frequency of immunization varies with type of vaccine and age immunization is initiated.

Taken from Ambulatory Child Health Care Protocols to be published by Sunbelt Medical Publishers in January 1992.

CHILD HEALTH SUPERVISION
6 MONTHS

EVALUATION/DIAGNOSTIC PROTOCOL
Subjective
Interval History. Which parents or significant others have accompanied the child? How is the baby described? How is the baby sleeping? Have there been illness or accidents? Are the eyes always straight? Has there been any reaction to immunizations?

General Nutritional. How is the baby nursing? Is he/she on formula? How much and how often? Has the baby started on solids? Are there any feeding difficulties? Vitamins? Fluoride? (Support programs WIC.)

Interval Key Family Checks. How is Mom's health? Are she and the infant on a regular schedule? Has either parent had a change of employment? Do the parents take time off? What are the child care arrangements? Have there been any other family changes? Is there tobacco, alcohol, or drug usage in the home?

Objective
Physical Examination. Vital signs (T and Wt, Wt%, Ht, Ht%, HC, HC%), general appearance, head (fontanelle), eyes (Hirschberg), cover/uncover test, ears (TMs), hearing, nose, oropharynx, neck, lungs, cardiovascular (femoral pulse), abdomen, genitalia, musculoskeletal, skin, lymph nodes, neurologic.

Development. Reaches? Coos? Rolls over? No head lag on pull to sit? Transfers? Sits with minimal support? Parent-child interaction?

Lab. Sickle prep, if indicated.

Assess the child's status.

Assess the family's status.

PLAN/MANAGEMENT PROTOCOL
General Measures/Anticipatory Guidance. Discuss sleep pattern, nutrition (introduction of solids and anticipate finger foods), elimination pattern.
   Discuss safety: car, safety-proofing, tub. Discuss play patterns, sleep patterns. Emphasize teaching appropriate stranger fear.
   Discuss teething. Discuss shoes. Distribute companion education and reference list.

Specific Measures. DPT #3, HIB.[1] Immunization education materials and releases.

Physician Consultation. At practitioner's discretion.

Follow-up Plan.

---

[1]Consult USPHS schedule as frequency of immunization varies with type of vaccine and age immunization is initiated.

Taken from Ambulatory Child Health Care Protocols to be published by Sunbelt Medical Publishers in January 1992.

CHILD HEALTH SUPERVISION
9 MONTHS

EVALUATION/DIAGNOSTIC PROTOCOL
Subjective

Interval History. Which parents or significant others have accompanied the child? How is the baby described? Has there been illness? Accidents?

General Nutritional. How is the baby nursing? Is he/she on formula? How much and how often? Has the baby started on solids? Is the baby feeding itself finger foods? Are there any feeding difficulties? Vitamins? Fluoride? (Support programs WIC.)

Interval Key Family Checks. Is there good child care support? Is the family in a comfortable routine? Has either parent had a change of employment? Has the social history of the family changed? Is the child in day care? Is there tobacco, alcohol, or drug usage in the home?

Objective

Physical Examination. Vital signs (T and Wt, Wt%, Ht, Ht%, HC, HC%), general appearance, head (fontanelle), eyes (Hirschberg), cover/uncover test, ears (TMs), hearing, nose, oropharynx, neck, lungs, cardiovascular, abdomen, genitalia, musculoskeletal, skin, lymph nodes, neurologic.

Development. Sits without support? Says "Mama" or "Dada"? Looks for a fallen object? Plays peek-a-boo? Pincer grasp? Stands holding on? Parent-child interaction?

Lab. Hct, UA, Pb if indicated.

Assess the child's status.

Assess the family's status.

PLAN/MANAGEMENT PROTOCOL

General Measures/Anticipatory Guidance. Discuss nutrition, weaning, use of cup. Discuss safety: falls, ingestions, Ipecac, car. Discuss play patterns. Discuss discipline (no spanking). Discuss daycare. Discuss separation anxiety. Distribute companion education and reference list.

Specific Measures. If unimmunized, begin immunizations. Immunization education materials.

Physician Consultation. At practitioner's discretion.

Follow-up Plan. _____ months.

Taken from Ambulatory Child Health Care Protocols to be published by Sunbelt Medical Publishers in January 1992.

CHILD HEALTH SUPERVISION
12 MONTHS

EVALUATION/DIAGNOSTIC PROTOCOL

Subjective

Interval History. Which parents or significant others have accompanied the child? How is the child described? Has there been illness? Accidents?

General Nutritional. Is the child still nursing? How many meals does the child eat per day? Is the diet reasonably varied and balanced? Any peculiarities (pica)? How much milk does the child drink? Are there any eating difficulties? Describe elimination pattern. Vitamins? Fluoride? Support programs?

Interval Key Family Checks. Is there good child care support? Is the family in a comfortable routine? Has either parent had a change of employment? Has the social history of the family changed? Are there safe and satisfactory child care arrangements? Is there tobacco, alcohol, or drug usage in the home?

Objective

Physical Examination. Vital signs (T and Wt, Wt%, Ht, Ht%, HC, HC%), general appearance, head (fontanelle), eyes (Hirschberg), cover/uncover test, ears (TMs), hearing, nose, oropharynx, neck, lungs, cardiovascular, abdomen, genitalia, musculoskeletal, skin, lymph nodes, neurologic.

Development. Bangs two blocks together? Specifies "Mama" or "Dada"? Initiates vocalizations? Understands "no"? Plays pat-a-cake? Cruises? Waves bye-bye? Stands alone 2-3"? Parent-child interaction?

Lab. TB.

Assess the child's status.

Assess the family's status.

PLAN/MANAGEMENT PROTOCOL

Measures/Anticipatory Guidance. Discuss dental care, use of toothbrush but no toothpaste. Discuss nutrition, weaning, appetite decrease. Discuss safety: falls, stairs, Ipecac, houseproofing. Discuss sleep patterns. Discuss play patterns, reading to child, picture books. Discuss discipline limits. Discuss separation problems. Distribute companion education and reference list.

Specific Measures. If unimmunized, begin immunizations. Immunization education materials.

Physician Consultation. At practitioner's discretion.

Follow-up Plan. _____ months.

Taken from <u>Ambulatory Child Health Care Protocols</u> to be published by Sunbelt Medical Publishers in January 1992.

CHILD HEALTH SUPERVISION
15 MONTHS

EVALUATION/DIAGNOSTIC PROTOCOL
Subjective
Interval History. Which parents or significant others have accompanied the child? How is the child described? Has there been illness? Accidents?

General Nutritional. How often is the child nursing? Is the child getting enough milk? Is the child eating a reasonably varied and balanced diet (avoiding junk foods)? Are there any mealtime problems? Vitamins? Fluoride?

Interval Key Family Checks. Do the parents agree on discipline? Is there good child care support? Is the family in a comfortable routine? Has either parent had a change of employment? Has the social history of the family changed? Are there safe and satisfactory child care arrangements? Is there tobacco, alcohol, or drug usage in the home?

Objective
Physical Examination. Vital signs (T and Wt, Wt%, Ht, Ht%, HC, HC%), general appearance, head (fontanelle), eyes (Hirschberg), cover/uncover test, ears (TMs), hearing, nose, oropharynx, neck, lungs, cardiovascular, abdomen, genitalia, musculoskeletal, skin, lymph nodes, neurologic.

Development. Stoops to recover toy? Can indicate wants without crying? Drinks from a cup with little spill? Crawls upstairs? Can roll or toss a ball? Walks well? Parent-child interaction?

Lab.

Assess the child's status.

Assess the family's status.

PLAN/MANAGEMENT PROTOCOL
General Measures/Anticipatory Guidance. Discuss nutrition: discuss discontinuing bottle, discontinuing pacifier. Discuss safety: aspiration, plastic bags. Discuss toilet training beliefs and readiness. Discuss discipline. Discuss play patterns, reading to child. Discuss day care, use of babysitters. Discuss tantrums. Distribute companion education and reference list.

Specific Measures. MMR, HIB.[1] Immunization education materials and releases.

Physician Consultation. At practitioner's discretion.

Follow-up Plan. _____ months.

---

[1]Consult USPHS schedule as frequency of immunization varies with type of vaccine and age immunization is initiated.

Taken from Ambulatory Child Health Care Protocols to be published by Sunbelt Medical Publishers in January 1992.

CHILD HEALTH SUPERVISION
18 MONTHS

EVALUATION/DIAGNOSTIC PROTOCOL

Subjective

Interval History. Which parents or significant others have accompanied the child? How is the child described? Has there been illness? Accidents? Pica? No past serious DPT reaction?

General Nutritional. How often is the child nursing? How much milk is the child drinking? Is the child eating a reasonably varied and balanced diet (avoiding junk foods)? Are there any mealtime problems? Is the child weaned to drink from a cup? Does the child use a spoon (spills some)? Vitamins? Fluoride? Are there any mealtime problems?

Interval Key Family Checks. Is there any sibling "rivalry"? Do the parents agree on discipline? Is there good child care support? Is the family in a comfortable routine? Has either parent had a change of employment? Has the social history of the family changed? Are there safe and satisfactory child care arrangements? Is there tobacco, alcohol, or drug usage in the home?

Objective

Physical Examination. Vital signs (T and Wt, Wt%, Ht, Ht%, HC, HC%), general appearance, head (fontanelle), eyes (Hirschberg), cover/uncover test, ears (TMs), hearing, nose, oropharynx, neck, lungs, cardiovascular, abdomen, genitalia, musculoskeletal, skin, lymph nodes, neurologic.

Development. Using three words or more other than "Mama" or "Dada"? Mimics household tasks? Stacks three blocks? Removes clothing? Walks up steps? Drinks from cup? Scribbles? Parent-child interaction?

Lab.

Assess the child's status.

Assess the family's status.

PLAN/MANAGEMENT PROTOCOL

General Measures/Anticipatory Guidance. Discuss moving the child from the crib to a bed. Discuss nutrition (no junk food, three meals per day). Confirm that stranger fear is common. Discuss the need for consistent expectations. Emphasize the need to praise good behavior often. Discuss "negativism": increasing child autonomy, expect the child's "no." Discuss thumbsucking, masturbation. Discuss toilet training. Discuss safety: car, house, outdoors, water. Discuss play patterns, reading to child. Distribute companion education and reference list.

Specific Measures. DPT #4, OPV #3. Immunization education materials.

Physician Consultation. At practitioner's discretion.

Follow-up Plan. _____ months.

Taken from _Ambulatory Child Health Care Protocols_ to be published by Sunbelt Medical Publishers in January 1992.

CHILD HEALTH SUPERVISION
24 MONTHS

EVALUATION/DIAGNOSTIC PROTOCOL

<u>Subjective</u>

Interval History. Which parents or significant others have accompanied the child? How is the child described? Has there been illness? Accidents?

General Nutritional. How is the child's diet? Does the child eat three meals per day (with little or no junk food/drink)? Has the child discontinued use of a bottle? Vitamins? Fluoride? Are there any mealtime problems?

Interval Key Family Checks. Do the parents agree on discipline? Is the family in a comfortable routine? Has either parent had a change of employment? Has the social history of the family changed? Are there safe and satisfactory child care arrangements? Are there any additions to the family's medical history? Is there tobacco, alcohol, or drug usage in the home?

<u>Objective</u>

Physical Examination. Vital signs (T and Wt, Wt%, Ht, Ht%, HC, HC%), general appearance, head (fontanelle), eyes (Hirschberg), cover/uncover test, ears (TMs), hearing, nose, oropharynx, neck, lungs, cardiovascular, abdomen, genitalia, musculoskeletal, skin, lymph nodes, neurologic.

Development. Simple household tasks? Knows body parts? Constructs 2-3 word sentences? Handles a spoon well? Walks down steps? Throws overhand? Parent-child interaction?

Lab. Usually Hct. Consider TB tine. Consider UA and culture.

<u>Assess</u> the child's status.

<u>Assess</u> the family's status.

PLAN/MANAGEMENT PROTOCOL

General Measures/Anticipatory Guidance. Discuss nutrition. Discuss dental care: daily use of toothbrush (no toothpaste). Discuss safety: car, house, outdoors, water, kitchen, sharp objects. Discuss play: reading books, watching TV. Discuss sleep (regular bedtime). Discuss toilet training. Discuss speech problems. Distribute companion education and reference list.

Specific Measures. If unimmunized, begin immunizations. Immunization education materials.

Physician Consultation. At practitioner's discretion.

Follow-up Plan. _____ months.

Taken from <u>Ambulatory Child Health Care Protocols</u> to be published by Sunbelt Medical Publishers in January 1992.

CHILD HEALTH SUPERVISION
5 YEARS

EVALUATION/DIAGNOSTIC PROTOCOL
Subjective
Interval History. Which parents or significant others have accompanied the child? How is the child described? Has the child been readied for school: Does the child feel good about herself/himself? Is the child's attention span adequate? Does the child separate easily? Does the child get along with others? Can the child follow directions? Has there been illness? Accidents?

General Nutritional. Is the child eating a reasonably balanced and varied diet? Vitamins? Fluoride?

Interval Key Family Checks. Is the family happy? Have there been any family changes? Are there any family history additions? Are the child care arrangements satisfactory? How is Mom's work or school? How is Dad's work or school? Is there tobacco, alcohol, or drug use in the home?

Objective
Physical Examination. Vital signs (T and Wt, Wt%, Ht, Ht%, HC, HC%), general appearance, head, eyes, fundi, ears (TMs), nose, teeth/gums, pharynx, neck, lungs, cardiovascular, abdomen, genitalia, musculoskeletal, skin, lymph nodes, neurologic.

Development. Heel-to-toe walk? Draws man (3-6 parts)? Opposites (2 of 3)? Dresses alone? Copies square, triangle? Parent-child inter action?

Lab. Visual acuity, hearing, Hct, TB, UA, if indicated.

Assess the child's status.

Assess the family's status.

PLAN/MANAGEMENT PROTOCOL
General Measures/Anticipatory Guidance. Discuss nutrition: snacks. Discuss exercise/fun. Discuss safety: cars, bike, outdoors, water, fire. Discuss learning telephone number and address. Discuss appropriate fear of strangers. Discuss school readiness. Emphasize dental care. Discuss discipline. Discuss home responsibilities. Distribute companion educational materials and reference list.

Specific Measures. DPT #5, OPV #4, MMR #2.[1] Immunization education materials and releases.

Physician Consultation. At practitioner's discretion.

Follow-up Plan. _____ months.

----

[1]Consult USPHS schedule as frequency of immunization varies with type of vaccine and age immunization is initiated.

Taken from Ambulatory Child Health Care Protocols to be published by Sunbelt Medical Publishers in January 1992.

CHILD HEALTH SUPERVISION
10 YEARS

EVALUATION/DIAGNOSTIC PROTOCOL
Subjective
Interval History. Which parents or significant others have accompanied the child? How is the child described? Are there any special concerns? Has there been illness? Accidents? Is the child physically active? Are there any problem habits? Is the child sleeping OK?

General Nutritional. Is the child's diet OK? Is the child's body image OK? Are the eating habits OK? Does the child have favorite foods?

Interval Key Family Checks. Have there been any marital changes, work changes, or recent moves? Is the after school care satisfactory? Are there any sibling problems? How are family interactions? Is there tobacco, alcohol, or drug use in the family?

Objective
Physical Examination. Vital signs (T and Wt, Wt%, Ht, Ht%, HC, HC%), general appearance, head, eyes, fundi, ears (TMs), nose, teeth/gums, pharynx, thyroid, breast, neck, lungs, cardiovascular, abdomen, genitalia (Tanner stage), scoliosis check, musculoskeletal, skin, lymph nodes, neurologic. Depression?

Development. School work OK? Peer interactions OK? Behavior OK? Best friend? Favorite TV show/magazine/movie/ad? Hobbies/ sports? Group activities? Tobacco use, alcohol, or drug use? Parent-child interaction?

Lab. Visual acuity, hearing. If indicated: Hct, TB, UA.

Assess the child's status.

Assess the family's status.

PLAN/MANAGEMENT PROTOCOL
General Measures/Anticipatory Guidance. Discuss nutrition: snacks, breakfast. Discuss exercise, regular bedtime. Emphasize dental hygiene and the need for exams. Discuss safety: cars, bike, outdoors, water. Discuss appropriate sex education. Discuss physical/sexual abuse concerns. Discuss the potential for tobacco/ETOH/drug abuse. Discuss the need to monitor television watching. Discuss home responsibilities/allowance. Discuss appropriate parenting: the need for rules, respect, communication. Distribute companion educational materials and reference list. The authors recommend "Human Sexuality: A Bibliography for Everyone" available from Sex Information and Education Council of the United States (SIECUS), 130 West 42 Street, New York, NY 10036.

Specific Measures. Immunization education materials.

Physician Consultation. At practitioner's discretion.

Follow-up Plan. _____ months.

Taken from Ambulatory Child Health Care Protocols to be published by Sunbelt Medical Publishers in January 1992.

CHILD HEALTH SUPERVISION
12 YEARS

EVALUATION/DIAGNOSTIC PROTOCOL

Subjective

Interval History. Which parents or significant others have accompanied the child? How is the child described? Who does the child live with? Has there been any interim illness? Accidents? Is the child sleeping OK? Appetite? Does the child exercise or participate in sports? How many hours per day are spent watching TV? Has she begun to menstruate? Any problems?

General Nutritional. Is the child's diet OK? Is the child's body image OK? Are the eating habits OK? Does the child have favorite foods?

Re Sports Participation. Is there chest pain on exertion? Have there been any localized injuries? Is exercise tolerance OK? Is there any family history of sudden death?

Interval Key Family Checks. Have there been any marital changes? Are family relationships OK? Is the after school care satisfactory? Is there tobacco, alcohol, or drug use in the family?

Objective

Physical Examination. Vital signs (T and Wt, Wt%, Ht, Ht%, HC, HC%), general appearance, head, eyes, fundi, ears (TMs), nose, teeth/gums, pharynx, thyroid, breast, neck, lungs, cardiovascular, abdomen, genitalia (Tanner stage), scoliosis check, musculoskeletal, skin, lymph nodes, neurologic. Depression?

Development. School work OK? What are the current grades? Any failures/repeats? Peer interactions OK? Behavior OK? Knowledge of pregnancy, STDs, safe sexual practice? Future plans, goals? Activities for fun? Tobacco use, alcohol, or drug use? Special boyfriends/girlfriends? Degree of intimacy? Parent-child interaction?

Lab. Visual acuity, hearing. If indicated: MMR with TB Tine; GC, Chlamydia, trich, and Pap; H&H; UA.

Assess the child's status.

Assess the family's status.

PLAN/MANAGEMENT PROTOCOL

General Measures/Anticipatory Guidance. Discuss need for good nutrition, exercise. Emphasize dental hygiene and the need for exams. Discuss use of seat belt/helmet. Discuss the potential for tobacco, alcohol, drug abuse. Discuss puberty/tampon use. Discuss how to approach sex education, birth control, and STDs. Discuss the need for breast or testicle self exam. Discuss the child's personal rights/ safety. Discuss peer and family relationships. Discuss appropriate parenting: the need for rules, respect, communication. Distribute companion educational materials and reference list. The authors recommend "Human Sexuality: A Bibliography for Everyone" available from Sex Information and Education Council of the United States (SIECUS), 130 West 42 Street, New York, NY 10036.

Specific Measures. Immunization education materials.

Physician Consultation. At practitioner's discretion.

Follow-up Plan. _____ months.

Taken from Ambulatory Child Health Care Protocols to be published by Sunbelt Medical Publishers in January 1992.

CHILD HEALTH SUPERVISION
14 YEARS

EVALUATION/DIAGNOSTIC PROTOCOL
Subjective
Interval History. Which parents or significant others have accompanied the child? How is the child described? Who does the child live with? Has there been any interim illness? Accidents? Is the child sleeping OK? Appetite? Does the child exercise or participate in sports? How many hours per day are spent watching TV? Are her menses OK?

General Nutritional. Is the child's diet OK? Is the child's body image OK? Are the eating habits OK? Does the child have favorite foods?

Re Sports Participation. Is there chest pain on exertion? Have there been any localized injuries? Is exercise tolerance OK? Is there any family history of sudden death?

Interval Key Family Checks. Have there been any marital changes? Are family relationships OK? Is there tobacco, alcohol, or drug use in the family?

Objective
Physical Examination. Vital signs (T and Wt, Wt%, Ht, Ht%, HC, HC%), general appearance, head, eyes, fundi, ears (TMs), nose, teeth/gums, pharynx, thyroid, breast, neck, lungs, cardiovascular, abdomen, genitalia (Tanner stage), scoliosis check, musculoskeletal, skin, lymph nodes, neurologic. Depression?

Development. School work OK? What are the current grades? Any failures/repeats? Peer interactions OK? Behavior OK? Knowledge of pregnancy, STDs, and safe sexual practice? Future plans, goals? Activities for fun? Tobacco use, alcohol, or drug use? Special boyfriends/girlfriends? Degree of intimacy? Parent-child interaction?

Lab. Visual acuity, hearing. If indicated: random cholesterol; UA; GC, chlamydia, trich, and Pap; H&H; dT if none x 10 years.

Assess the child's status.

Assess the family's status.

PLAN/MANAGEMENT PROTOCOL
General Measures/Anticipatory Guidance. Discuss need for good nutrition, exercise. Emphasize dental hygiene and the need for exams. Discuss use of seat belt/helmet. Discuss the potential for tobacco, alcohol, drug abuse. Discuss puberty/tampon use. Discuss how to approach sex education, birth control, and STDs. Discuss the need for breast or testicle self exam. Discuss the child's personal rights/ safety. Discuss peer and family relationships. Discuss appropriate parenting: the need for rules, respect, communication. Distribute companion educational materials and reference list. The authors recommend "Human Sexuality: A Bibliography for Everyone" available from Sex Information and Education Council of the United States (SIECUS), 130 West 42 Street, New York, NY 10036.

Specific Measures. Immunization education materials.

Physician Consultation. At practitioner's discretion.

Follow-up Plan. _____ months.

Taken from Ambulatory Child Health Care Protocols to be published by Sunbelt Medical Publishers in January 1992.

CHILD HEALTH SUPERVISION
16 YEARS

EVALUATION/DIAGNOSTIC PROTOCOL
<u>Subjective</u>
Interval History. Which parents or significant others have accompanied the child? How is the child described? Who does the child live with? Has there been any interim illness? Accidents? Is the child sleeping OK? Appetite? Does the child exercise or participate in sports? How many hours per day are spent watching TV? Are her menses OK? Driver's license?

General Nutritional. Is the child's diet OK? Is the child's body image OK? Are the eating habits OK? Does the child have favorite foods?

Re Sports Participation. Is there chest pain on exertion? Have there been any localized injuries? Is exercise tolerance OK? Is there any family history of sudden death?

Interval Key Family Checks. Have there been any marital changes? Are family relationships OK? Is there tobacco, alcohol, or drug use in the family?

<u>Objective</u>
Physical Examination. Vital signs (T and Wt, Wt%, Ht, Ht%, HC, HC%), general appearance, head, eyes, fundi, ears (TMs), nose, teeth/gums, pharynx, thyroid, breast, neck, lungs, cardiovascular, abdomen, pelvic exam if indicated, genitalia (Tanner stage), scoliosis check, musculoskeletal, skin, lymph nodes, neurologic. Depression?

Development. School work OK? What are the current grades? Any failures/repeats? Peer interactions OK? Behavior OK? Knowledge of pregnancy, STDs, and safe sexual practice? Job, future plans? Activities for fun? Tobacco use, alcohol, or drug use? Special boyfriends/girlfriends? Sexual relationships? Parent-child interaction?

Lab. Visual acuity, hearing. If indicated: random cholesterol; UA; GC, chlamydia, trich, and Pap; H&H; dT if none x 10 years.

<u>Assess</u> the child's status.

<u>Assess</u> the family's status.

PLAN/MANAGEMENT PROTOCOL
General Measures/Anticipatory Guidance. Discuss need for good nutrition, exercise. Emphasize dental hygiene and the need for exams. Discuss use of seat belt/helmet. Discuss the potential for tobacco, alcohol, drug abuse. Discuss drinking and driving. Discuss how to approach sex education, birth control, and STDs. Discuss the need for breast or testicle self exam. Discuss the need for safety: sex, birth control. Discuss how to "see through" deceptive ads. Discuss peer and family relationships. Discuss appropriate parenting: the need for rules, respect, communication. Distribute companion educational materials and reference list. The authors recommend "Human Sexuality: A Bibliography for Everyone" available from <u>Sex Information and Education Council of the United States</u> (<u>SIECUS</u>), 130 West 42 Street, New York, NY 10036.

Specific Measures. Immunization education materials.

Physician Consultation. At practitioner's discretion.

Follow-up Plan. _____ months.

Taken from <u>Ambulatory Child Health Care Protocols</u> to be published by Sunbelt Medical Publishers in January 1992.

Preventive Health Care, Adults

YEARS: 21 22 23 24 25 26 27 28 29 30 31 32 33 34 35 36 37 38 39 40 41 42 43 44 45 46 47 48 49 50 51 52 53 54 55 56 57 58 59 60 61 62 63 64 65 66 67 68 69 70

SUBJECTIVE
- Complete initial interview Hx
- Update Hx

OBJECTIVE
- Complete/interval PEx
- Ht, Wt, P., BP, R
- Thyroid Ex Women
- Breast Ex Women
- Pelvic Women
- Rectal
- Visual Scr./Glaucoma Scr.
- Hearing Scr.

LAB
- Pap
- Hct Women
- Mammography
- U/A
- Hct Men
- Guaiac X6
- Flex Sig
- Tb Test
- Chemistry Panel
- Thyroid Panel
- Lipid Panel
- RPR/VDRL
- EKG
- Pulmonary Function/CXR
- GXT

ANTICIPATORY GUIDANCE
- Prudent Diet
- Exercise Regime
- Alcohol/Drug/Tobacco Use
- Safe Sex/Sex
- Seatbelt
- Self Exam/Warning Signs

THERAPY
- dT
- Influenza

Preventive Health Care, Adults

YEARS: 21 22 23 24 25 26 27 28 29 30 31 32 33 34 35 36 37 38 39 40 41 42 43 44 45 46 47 48 49 50 51 52 53 54 55 56 57 58 59 60 61 62 63 64 65 66 67 68 69 70

SUBJECTIVE
- Complete initial interview Hx
- Update Hx

OBJECTIVE
- Complete/interval PEx
- Ht, Wt, P, BP, R
- Thyroid Ex Women
- Breast Ex Women
- Pelvic Women
- Rectal
- Visual Scr./Glaucoma Scr.
- Hearing Scr.

LAB
- Pap
- Hct Women
- Mammography
- U/A
- Hct Men
- Guaiac X6
- Flex Sig
- Tb Test
- Chemistry Panel
- Thyroid Panel
- Lipid Panel
- RPR/VDRL
- EKG
- Pulmonary Function/CXR
- GXT

ANTICIPATORY GUIDANCE
- Prudent Diet
- Exercise Regime
- Alcohol/Drug/Tobacco Use
- Safe Sex/Sex
- Seatbelt
- Self Exam/Warning Signs

THERAPY
- dT
- Influenza

Cardiac or Respiratory Arrest, Infants

EVALUATION/DIAGNOSTIC PROTOCOL
Subjective
History.

Objective
Physical Exam. A. Is Airway Obstructed?
                   B. Are there Respirations?
                   C. Is there a Pulse?

PLAN/MANAGEMENT PROTOCOL
General Measures. SUMMON EMERGENCY MEDICAL SERVICES.

Specific Measures.   2 RESCUERS
                   Should be Qualified in Basic Cardiac Life Support

Open **Airway** without neck hyperextension

Rescue **Breathing** 1 breath every 3 seconds (mouth-to-mouth or consider mouth-to-mouth or bag-valve mouth)

                                               Ratio 5:1
Circulatory Support 100 Chest compressions every 1 minute

Physician Consultation. Mandatory.

Referral.

Immediate Transfer. To _____.

Follow-up Plan.

                                        Initials   Date
                                        Physician
                                        ARNP

Cardiac or Respiratory Arrest, Children

EVALUATION/DIAGNOSTIC PROTOCOL
<u>Subjective</u>
History.

<u>Objective</u>
Physical Exam.   A.   Is Airway Obstructed?
                 B.   Are there Respirations?
                 C.   Is there a Pulse?

PLAN/MANAGEMENT PROTOCOL
General Measures.   SUMMON EMERGENCY MEDICAL SERVICES

Specific Measures.   2 RESCUERS
               Should be Qualified in Basic Cardiac Life Support

Open Airway

Rescue Breathing   1 breath every 4 seconds (mouth-to-mouth or consider mouth-to-mouth or bag-valve mouth)

                                             Ratio 5:1
Circulatory Support 80-100 Chest compressions every 1 minute

Physician Consultation.   Mandatory.

Referral.

Immediate Transfer.   To _____.

Follow-up Plan.

                                               Initials   Date
                                               Physician
                                               ARNP

Cardiac or Respiratory Arrest, Adults

EVALUATION/DIAGNOSTIC PROTOCOL
Subjective
History.

Objective
Physical Exam.   A.   Is Airway Obstructed?
                     B.   Are there Respirations?
                     C.   Is there a Pulse?

PLAN/MANAGEMENT PROTOCOL
General Measures. SUMMON EMERGENCY MEDICAL SERVICES

Specific Measures.   2 RESCUERS
                 Should be Qualified in Basic Cardiac Life Support

Open Airway

Rescue Breathing 1 breath every 5 seconds (mouth-to-mouth or consider mouth-to-mouth or bag-valve mouth)

                                                 Ratio 5:1
Circulatory Support 80 Chest compressions every 1 minute

Physician Consultation. Mandatory.

Referral.

Immediate Transfer. To _____.

Follow-up Plan.

                                               Initials   Date
                                               Physician
                                               ARNP

Acute Chest Pain

EVALUATION/DIAGNOSTIC PROTOCOL
Subjective
History. Description of the pain, severity, quality, aggravating and alleviating circumstances, duration of each episode, location, radiation, and accompanying symptomatology. Are there predisposing factors: habits (smoking), family history, situational, injury? Are there underlying conditions: hypertension, diabetes, hyperlipidemia, gastrointestinal disease? Note: angina pectoris/myocardial ischemic pain occurs with exertion (or stress) and lasts at least several minutes but not longer than ten. (See Angina Pectoris). Persistent "pressure" may represent infarct and is an emergency requiring **immediate transfer**. Costochondritis and other musculoskeletal causes usually are localized with exacerbations due to positioning and various motions.

Objective
Physical Examination. General appearance, vital signs, chest, complete cardio-vascular and abdominal exam. Costochondral junction or other discrete area tenderness is most consistent with musculoskeletal etiology.

Lab. EKG, chest x-ray, and _____.

Assessment is directed toward differentiating the acute emergency from non-emergent chest pain. **Differential Diagnosis** includes myocardial infarction, pulmonary embolus, aortic dissection, pneumothorax, pericarditis and for that matter any history compatible with unstable angina are life-threatening and if being considered then **physician consultation and/or immediate transfer** is/are indicated. Other possibilities include pleuritis (also, see Pneumonia, Adult), esophageal spasm, other gastointestinal (see Peptic Ulcer Disease) and intra-abdominal causes (see Abdominal Pain, Adults), costochondritis or other musculo-skeletal pain (and also see Herpes Zoster). **Complications** are potentially so serious that unless you are certain the cause is amongst the last few diagnoses discussed then physician consultation is necessary.

PLAN/MANAGEMENT PROTOCOL
General Measures are determined by the suspected etiology.

Specific Measures are determined by the specific etiology.

Physician Consultation is absolutely necessary if not diagnostically certain the pain is either musculoskeletal or a non-emergent G.I. cause in origin.

Referral.

Immediate Transfer if suspicious of life-threatening cause, to _____.

Follow-up Plan.

Initials   Date
Physician
ARNP

Seizures, Children

EVALUATION/DIAGNOSTIC PROTOCOL
Subjective
History. Detailed medical history, including birth history. Emphasis is on the recent history (febrile episode?) circumstances surrounding the seizure, preceding (prodromal), accompanying (focality) and subsequent (postictal) symptoms. Previous or family history. Predisposing circumstances or underlying conditions. Has the child been on any medications?

Objective
Physical Examination. Complete physical exam with attention to a thorough age appropriate neurologic and developmental exam.

Lab must be individualized consider CBC, chemistry panel (include glucose, ammonia, calcium, BUN, creatinine), toxicology screen urine and/or blood. If known epileptic, the measure level of anticonvulsants currently taking; also consider levels of other medications (i.e., theophylline). If meningitis is a possibility, then refer/do **lumbar puncture and appropriate CSF studies**. In certain settings consider skull films, CAT of the head, EEG.

Assessment is directed at the etiology, **always consult attending**. **Differential Diagnosis**. Excepting the immediate neonatal period the most common cause of seizures is a febrile convulsion (a diagnosis of exclusion). The more significant **emergent** causes are meningitis, trauma, accidental ingestion, metabolic imbalance, tumor. Other common causes include idiopathic, familial, and breathholding. **Complications** are related to the etiology but also include those common to seizures such as aspiration, self-injury, prologed hypoxia and coma.

PLAN/MANAGEMENT PROTOCOL
ACTIVELY SEIZING
General Measures. As most seizures are self-limited, your initial response is to protect the patient from self-harm. **Maintain the airway** and place the child in a location where the convulsive motions won't allow injury. In the young child institute antipyretic measures such as acetaminophen suppository. Summon physician but stay with the child. For episodes approaching 10 minutes call emergency medical services.

Specific Measures. Should be instituted by attending physician. Administer oxygen, suction as needed, begin IV Ringer's Lactate.
Establishing protocols for medications depends on nurse practitioner training.
Consider IV anticonvulsant _____*(MIS).

As an alternative if physician not on premises, establish additional guidelines.

RECENT SEIZURE
General Measures. If initial event, then consult physician. Do review with patient and family the necessity of diagnostic evaluation and/or referral, general precautions , as well as specific observations and precautions should seizure recur. Give reinforcing educational literature and consider referral to Epilepsy Foundation.

Specific Measures. Prescribe or adjust anticonvulsant after consultation.

Physician Consultation is mandatory for all active or recent seizures.

Referral per attending physician to neurologist _____.

Immediate Transfer when indicated to_____.

Follow-up Plan depends entirely on the etiology.

	Initials	Date
* unless allergic, contraindicated,	Physician	
or pregnant/lactating	ARNP	

Seizures, Adults

EVALUATION/DIAGNOSTIC PROTOCOL
Subjective
History. General medical history with emphasis on the circumstances surrounding the seizure, preceding (prodromal), accompanying (focality) and subsequent (postictal) symptoms. Previous or family history. Predisposing circumstances or underlying conditions. Any medications OTC or prescribed?

Objective
Physical Examination. Complete physical exam with thorough neurologic exam (include mental status screen).

Lab. Consider CBC, chemistry panel (include glucose, calcium, magnesium, BUN, creatinine), alcohol, toxicology screen urine and/or blood. If known epileptic, then measure level of anticonvulsants currently taking; also consider levels of other medications (i.e., theophylline). If meningitis is a possibility then refer/do lumbar puncture and appropriate CSF studies. Consider skull films, CAT of the head, EEG.

Assessment is directed at the etiology. Differential Diagnosis includes the various epilepsies (amongst those being treated causes include withdrawal from medications, inadequate dosing, intercurrent illness, other drugs and alcohol), drug toxicity or withdrawal, alcohol, intracranal mass, injury, meningitis, metaboloic derangement (hypoglycemic reaction most commonly), hypoxia/anoxia, cerebrovascular event. Complications are related to the etiology but also include self-injury, aspiration, anoxia and coma.

PLAN/MANAGEMENT PROTOCOL
ACTIVELY SEIZING
General Measures. As most seizures are self-limited, your initial response is to protect the patient from self-harm. Maintain the airway, suction and administer oxygen as needed. Place the patient in a location where the convulsive motions won't allow injury. Summon physician but stay with the patient. For episodes approaching 10 minutes call emergency medical services.

Specific Measures. While instituting general measures obtain blood for tests then begin IV Ringer's Lactate, followed immediately by 50 ml of D50.
Consider IV anticonvulsant _____ *(MIS).

RECENT SEIZURE
General Measures. If initial event, then consult attending physician. Do review with patient and family the necessity of diagnostic evaluation and/or referrral, general precautions, as well as specific observations and general precautions should seizure recur. Give reinforcing literature and referral to Epilepsy Foundation.

Specific Measures. Prescribe or adjust anticonvulsant dosage after consultation.

Physician Consultation for all active or recent seizures.

Referral as advised by attending to neurologist _____.

Immediate Transfer for status epilepticus to _____.

Follow-up Plan is always individualized. Review emergency plans with patient.

	Initials	Date
* unless allergic, contraindicated,	Physician	
or pregnant/lactating	ARNP	

Accidental Ingestions, Infants and Children

EVALUATION/DIAGNOSTIC PROTOCOL

Subjective

History of the circumstances surrounding the ingestion. Try to determine the exact amount of the ingestion as well as the exact ingestant. Know the time of the occurrence. **This is an emergency.** Is the child on other medications? Obtain personal history of accidents. How was this child supervised (consider neglect). Is this a family in turmoil or undergoing change(ingestions are more common in these settings). In children of school age consider this may be a suicide attempt.

Objective

Physical Examination. Complete physical exam.

Lab. If necessary, this patient may be better managed in a hospital emergency room.

Assessment is to determine the potential for the ingestant(s) to cause death or result in serious injury. Phone the nearest Poison Control Center _____. **Complications** depend on the ingestant.

PLAN/MANAGEMENT PROTOCOL

General Measures. Remind the family that the young child should be closely supervised. Potential poisons should be removed from the child's environment. The older child must be taught what things are dangerous to eat or drink. A child who has had one accidental ingestion statistically has a 50% chance of another.

Consequently, every effort should be made to limit the number of potential poisons in the home and lock up known poisons, including those which most commonly cause death or serious injury; all medicines (not just prescriptions but also OTC drugs including aspirin, acetaminophen, iron containing pills), liquid or granulated drain cleaner, dish-washer detergents, powdered bleach, spot remover, nail polish remover, insecticides, herbicides, paints and paint thiners, gasoline, oils and kerosene. Children must be taught not to put plant stuffs in their mouths especially berries, seeds and mushrooms.

Specific Measures are to induce emesis if not contraindicated for the ingestant (strong acid, strong alkali, some hydrocarbons) or by decreased level of consciousness. Give *syrup of ipecac 15 ml folowed by 4-8 ounces of water.

Physician Consultation. On all patients.

Immediate Transfer or dispatch Emergency Medical Services to the patient when circumstances warrant intervention and ipecac not on hand.

Follow-up Plan. Usually not necessary. Child should resume nursing or have clear liquids only until well tolerated.

Initials   Date

* unless allergic, contraindicated,   Physician
or pregnant/lactating   ARNP

Anaphylaxis, Infants and Children

EVALUATION/DIAGNOSTIC PROTOCOL
Subjective
History. This is a medical emergency. **Focus immediately on treatment**. When able, ascertain likely etiology, bee sting, wasp sting, hornet sting, fire ant bite, adverse drug reaction (oral or injectible), occasionally food or other ingestant.

Objective
Physical Examination. General appearance (pallor), vital signs (decreased blood pressure, increased pulse), respiratory distress.

Lab. None.

Assessment. Note: This is a life-threatening emergency, if patient has severe bronchospasm, airway obstruction, cyanosis.

PLAN/MANAGEMENT PROTOCOL
General Measures. Summon Emergency Medical Services.

Specific Measures.
Aqueous epinephrine 1:1000 0.01 ml/kg (to maximum dose of 0.2 ml) subcutanteously.
    Establish I.V. route, Ringer's Lactate.
    Administer oxygen and maintain airway.
    Consider hydrocortisone, 10 mg/kg I.V.P.
    Consider diphenhydramine*, 0.5-1.0 mg/kg I.V.

Physician Consultation. Immediate.

Referral.

Immediate Transfer. To _____.

Follow-up Plan.

		Initials	Date
* unless allergic, contraindicated, or pregnant/lactating	Physician ARNP		

Anaphylaxis, Adults

EVALUATION/DIAGNOSTIC PROTOCOL

Subjective

History. This is a medical emergency. Focus immediately on treatment. When able, ascertain likely etiology, bee sting, wasp sting, hornet sting, fire ant bite, averse drug reaction (oral or injectible), occasionally food or other ingestant.

Objective

Physical Examination. General appearance (pallor), vital signs (decreased blood pressure, increased pulse), respiratory distress.

Lab. None.

Assessment. Note: This is a life-threatening emergency, if patient has severe bronchospasm, airway obstruction, cyanosis.

PLAN/MANAGEMENT PROTOCOL

General Measures. Summon Emergency Medical Services.

Specific Measures. Aqueous epinephrine 1:1000 <u>0.3-0.5 ml</u> subcutaneously.
    Establish I.V. route, normal saline or Ringer's lactate.
    Administer oxygen and maintain airway.
    Consider hydrocortisone, <u>500 mg</u> I.V. push.
    Consider diphenhydramine*, <u>50 mg</u> I.V.

Physician Consultation. Immediate.

Referral.

Immediate Transfer. To _____.

Follow-up Plan.

		Initials	Date

* unless allergic, contraindicated,   Physician
or pregnant/lactating   ARNP

Insect Sting, Local Reaction (Children and Adults)

EVALUATION/DIAGNOSTIC PROTOCOL

<u>Subjective</u>

History. Course and onset of symptoms. What insect, when, what treatments preceded patient's arrival?

<u>Objective</u>

Physical Examination. General appearance, vital signs, complete skin exam. (If signs of diffuse reaction (see <u>Insect Sting, Diffuse Reaction</u>). Always examine face, mouth, and auscultate chest for signs of diffuse reaction and pending anaphylaxis.

Lab.

<u>Assess</u> that this is a local reaction. (If diffuse, see that section and <u>review anaphylaxis</u> protocol).

PLAN/MANAGEMENT PROTOCOL

General Measures. Apply ice water compresses to the affected area. Keep cool and at minimal activity level. Consider bathing in cool to tepid bath with addition of colloidal oatmeal.
     Encourage the patient or parent to eliminate exposure to the offending insect.

Specific Measures.
Consider topical corticosteroid _____ *(MIS)

and/or

Consider Rx for oral antihistamine _____ *(MIS)

Physician Consultation. Consider if signs of diffuse reaction, lack of response to therapy, prolonged history of symptoms, or recurrence with treatment failures.

Referral.

Immediate Transfer. If developing anaphylaxis, summon emergency medical services.

Follow-up Plan. In _____ day(s) if persistent symptoms, sooner if worse. Be sure to caution patient about signs and symptoms of diffuse reaction and anaphylaxis and the need for immediate attention.

	Initials	Date
* unless allergic, contraindicated, or pregnant/lactating	Physician ARNP	

Insect Sting, Diffuse Reaction (Children and Adults)

EVALUATION/DIAGNOSTIC PROTOCOL

Subjective

History. Course and onset of symptoms. What insect, when, what treatments preceded patient's arrival?

Objective

Physical Examination. General appearance, vital signs (hypotension), complete skin exam (urticaria, angioedema, general pallor). Always examine face, mouth, and auscultate chest for signs of diffuse reaction and pending anaphylaxis.

Lab. Consider testing for venom sensitivity by _____.

Assess that this is no longer just a local reaction, (see Anaphylaxis).

PLAN/MANAGEMENT PROTOCOL

General Measures. Keep cool and at minimal activity level. Consider bathing in cool to tepid bath with addition of colloidal oatmeal.

Encourage the patient or parent to eliminate exposure to the offending insect. Discuss the possibility of instituting or referring for desensitization to the insect venom. Review signs and symptoms that indicate worsening reactions. Make provisions for family member or patient to use epinephrine kit.

Specific Measures.

ACUTE REACTION

Consider aqueous epinephrine 1:1000 <u>0.01 ml/kg</u> subcutaneously (<u>see Anaphylaxsis</u>).

Consider corticosteroid* IM or IV_____.

Consider antihistamine* IM or IV_____.

THEN

Consider Rx for oral antihistamine _____*(MIS)

and/or

Consider Rx for oral corticosteroid _____*(MIS).

Physician Consultation. Consider if a diffuse reaction, lack of response to therapy, prolonged history of symptoms, or recurrence with treatment failures.

Referral.

Immediate Transfer. If developing anaphylaxis, summon emergency medical services.

Follow-up Plan. In _____ day(s) if persistent symptoms, sooner if worse.

	Initials	Date
* unless allergic, contraindicated, or pregnant/lactating	Physician ARNP	

Animal Bites, Non-Venomous

EVALUATION/DIAGNOSTIC PROTOCOL

Subjective

History. Circumstances of the bite and whether it was provoked or unprovoked and by what type of animal, domestic or wild (raccoon, bat, fox, skunk). Is there rabies locally? Is the animal captured or dead? Has bite been reported? What symptoms is the patient complaining about?

Objective

Physical Examination. General appearance, vital signs, wound description. If puncture or penetrating injury in a non-clothed area there is increased risk for rabies. Remainder of exam is directed at the other areas of injury.

Lab.

Assess amount of tissue damage and risk for rabies.

PLAN/MANAGEMENT PROTOCOL

General Measures. Cleanse wound with Zephiran or Betadine. Small puncture wounds should be left open and gently irrigated. Larger lacerations should be repaired (see Minor Lacerations). Tetanus toxoid booster if indicated. Notify local law enforcement or animal control officer.

Specific Measures. If serious risk for rabies, begin current U.S. Public Health rabies protocol.

Consider antibiotic prophylaxis Rx _____*(MIS).

Physician Consultation. If rabies is a possibility or if significant wound and sensitive or cosmetically significant area. Also, if litigation a possibility.

Referral to be considered for face and hand injuries to plastic surgeon and for other injuries to the appropriate specialist.

Immediate Transfer as indicated, to _____.

Follow-up Plan. No follow-up necessary for minor bite unless signs or symptoms of infection. Otherwise, follow-up dictated by degree of repair and for rabies immunization.

	Initials	Date
* unless allergic, contraindicated,	Physician	
or pregnant/lactating	ARNP	

Human Bites

EVALUATION/DIAGNOSTIC PROTOCOL

Subjective

History. Circumstances of the bite, biter and bitten (patient) full names, (if minors then the names of supervising adults), date, time and where incident happened. For adults or teens whether provoked assault and corroborating witnesses. Assault or suspected abuse should be reported to local authorities.

Objective

Physical Examination. General appearance, vital signs, wound location and description. Abrasion, puncture or penetrating injury?

Lab. Consider wound culture. Consider hepatitis screen, HIV, etc., to establish status for future reference.

Assess amount of tissue damage and risk for transmittable diseases. Complications are secondary infection, functional impairment and cosmetic disfigurement.

PLAN/MANAGEMENT PROTOCOL

General Measures. Cleanse wound with Zephiran or Betadine. Small puncture wounds should be left open and gently irrigated. Larger lacerations should be repaired. Tetanus toxoid booster if indicated. Notify local authorities.

Specific Measures. Consider antibiotic prophylaxis Rx _____*(MIS).

Physician Consultation. If litigation a possibility because of assault or suspected abuse or if significant wound or if in sensitive or cosmetically significant area.

Referral. Should be considered for facial and hand and finger injuries to plastic surgeon.

Immediate Transfer. As indicated to _____.

Follow-up Plan. No follow-up necessary for minor bite unless signs or symptoms of infection. Otherwise, follow-up dictated by degree of repair and need for follow-up testing for transmittable disorders.

		Initials Date
* unless allergic, contraindicated,	Physician	
or pregnant/lactating	ARNP	

Minor Lacerations

EVALUATION/DIAGNOSTIC PROTOCOL

Subjective

History. Obtain details of circumstances surrounding the injury. Any underlying conditions that might have predisposed the patient toward the injury? Any medications (over-the-counter, prescription, illicit) being used? If head wound, then document any alteration in sensorium (see Head Trauma).

Objective

Physical Examination. General appearance, vital signs, wound location and description with attention to whether or not there is any functional impairment. Consider diagramming the anatomic location showing, also the wound pre- and post-repair when the you record the physical examination.

Lab. Usually none.

Assessment. Characterize the wound as abrasion (with or without embedded foreign matter), simple laceration, avulsion/flap-type laceration. Do not close lacerations that are more than 6 hours old. **Differentiate** minor lacerations from the more significant injury with ligament, tendon or nerve damage. **Complications** are secondary wound infection and/or disruption of repair.

PLAN/MANAGEMENT PROTOCOL

General Measures. Soak in _____*(MIS).
      Cleanse with _____*(MIS), then explore to be certain all foreign material is removed. Debride appropriately, then consider irrigation or recleansing.

Specific Measures. For abrasions and very minor lacerations, consider closing with adhesive strips or patch _____.
      For suturable wounds, anesthetize appropriately with _____ _____, then explore the wound prior to closure.
      Close with _____ _____ along relaxed skin tension lines.
      Tetanus prophylaxis,* and for animal bites rabies precautions and/or rabies prophylaxis.

Physician Consultation. For all wounds over 6 hours old, penetrating or puncture wounds, those resulting from an altercation, those suspicious of or reflecting abuse or neglect, those by a contaminated object, those occurring in non-chlorinated fresh water, those on the face for adults and children, those on the hands, those longer than one centimeter in young children, or those where you are not confident that repair will be simple and easy.

Referral. Consider referring facial wounds to plastic surgeon (in particular if desired by patient or parent), eyelid and wounds to plastic surgeon or ophthalmologist, wounds with functional impairment to the appropriate plastic or orthopedic surgeon.

Immediate Transfer. Indicated if suspicion of internal organ damage, functional impairment (in some instances), and for bleeding not easily brought under control.

Follow-up Plan. Recheck as indicated in _____ day(s). Suture removal as indicated in _____ days. Recheck sooner if signs or symptoms of infection. Be certain to review these with the patient as well as suture care measures and dressing change instructions.

	Initials	Date
* unless allergic, contraindicated, or pregnant/lactating	Physician ARNP	

Minor Burns

EVALUATION/DIAGNOSTIC PROTOCOL

<u>Subjective</u>

History. Obtain detailed history of the circumstances surrounding the injury and what, if any, first aid measures have been employed. Determine whether there are predisposing circumstances or underlying conditions that resulted in the injury.

<u>Objective</u>

Physical Examination. General appearance, vital signs, complete skin exam. Be certain to describe the burns both as to degree and location. (Employ rule of 9's.) First-degree burns--simple erythema, painful to the touch. Second-degree burns--vesicle or blister formation (partial-thickness). Third-degree burns--may be charred and hard or may be pale to white. In some situations, subcutaneous fat may be visible.

Lab. None.

<u>Assess</u> degree and percent of surface area. Consider the patient's palm to equal 1% of the body surface area. **Complications** are secondary infections and restrictive scars.

<u>PLAN/MANAGEMENT PROTOCOL</u>

General Measures. Immerse the burned area in ice-cold water. Discuss prevention.

Specific Measures. Depending on degree, percent of body surface involved, and/or location, consider analgesic therapy with _____*(MIS).

    Gently clean affected area. Debride only ruptured blisters, otherwise do not disturb others.
    Cover with <u>silver sulfadizine cream</u> or _____, then a non-adherent dressing covered with bulky dressing.
    If necessary, institute appropriate tetanus prophylaxis.*

Physician Consultation. On all infants. Also on all third-degree burns. On burns as a result of suspected or known assault, abuse or neglect. Additionally, consult for all burns on the face, genitals or that involve considerable portion of either hand.

Referral.

Immediate Transfer. Should be considered for any third-degree burn greater than 4.5% of the body surface, any child with second-degree burns greater than 9%, and any adult with second-degree burns greater than 18%.

Follow-up Plan. Recheck the patient and redress the burn every _____ day(s) until satisfactorily healed or until family member or patient can be taught to redress the burn between follow-up visits.

	Initials	Date
* unless allergic, contraindicated, or pregnant/lactating Physician		
ARNP		

Head Trauma

EVALUATION/DIAGNOSTIC PROTOCOL

Subjective

History. Review in detail the circumstances of injury. Then, ascertain the sequence of neurologic and any other symptoms, with particular attention to level of consciousness, cognitive function, change, and focal signs. Are there predisposing conditions or circumstances, underlying medical conditions? Note any and all medications.

Objective

Physical Examination. General appearance, vital signs, head, complete eye, complete ENT, neck, and complete neurologic exam. (If altered level of consciousness, signs of intercranial injury including hypotension, Battle's sign, hemotympanum, CSF leakage either from ears or nose, or focal neurologic findings, then immediate transfer is indicated.)

Lab. Do/don't consider skull films and/or CAT of the head.

Assess severity or potential severity of the injury. **Differential Diagnosis** includes concussion syndrome, subdural hematoma, epidural hemorrhage, skull fracture. **Complications.** Any evidence of major head injury requires **immediate** transfer as increased intracranial pressure is life-threatening. Other complications relate to presense of underlying pathology.

PLAN/MANAGEMENT PROTOCOL

General Measures.
   1. Explain to patient and/or parents the term concussion and about the need for concern after head trauma (give head injury instruction sheet). Apply ice pack to site of contusion.
   2. If nausea, go to clear liquid diet for _____ hours.
   3. If headache, treat only with acetaminophen at appropriate dose for age and/or weight. Patient should be kept resting, preferably lying flat.
   4. The patient should be observed closely every _____ hour(s) for the next 24 hours, including awakening at night, for those things listed on the head injury instruction sheet.

Specific Measures. Never give narcotic analgesics or other drugs which may hamper assessment of developing complications.

Physician Consultation. For all patients with head trauma not obviously minor.

Referral. To neurosurgeon _____.

Immediate Transfer. To _____.

Follow-up Plan. As indicated by patient's condition or sooner as on Head Injury Sheet.

		Initials Date
* unless allergic, contraindicated, or pregnant/lactating	Physician ARNP	

Non-Traumatic Abdominal Pain (Children)

EVALUATION/DIAGNOSTIC PROTOCOL
<u>Subjective</u>
History. Detailed description of pain beginning with characteristics and location at onset and subsequently. Detail aggravating and alleviating factors, radiating and accompanying symptomatology, previous similar symptomatology.

<u>Objective</u>
Physical Examination. General appearance, vital signs, ENT, chest, abdomen, and rectal (if indicated).

Lab. Stool guaiac, stool obtained on rectal exam and UA. Hold for C&S. (If positive or suspicious, see <u>Urinary Tract Infection in Children</u>.) Consider stool for ova and parasites, stool for enteric pathogen. And, if suspected acute abdomen, consider CBC, flat and upright abdominal x-ray series.

<u>Assessment</u>. Try to decide whether or not this is an acute abdomen. It is most common for pain to be the result of viral, bacterial or protozoal gastroenteritis or from intestinal parasites. (See <u>Gastroenteritis in Children</u>.) Consider also medication or other ingestants. In the older child, school phobia is a diagnosis of exclusion. **Differential diagnosis** should include causes of acute abdomen, appendicitis at any age, malrotation or volvulus under 1 month of age, intussusception under 2 years of age. These are emergencies. Consider also pain as a result of medications, peptic ulcer disease, and accidental ingestions (see also <u>Abdominal Pain [Adults]</u>). **Complications** depend on etiology.

PLAN/MANAGEMENT PROTOCOL
General Measures. Review with parents likely and suspected diagnosis and particular signs or symptoms of acute abdominal conditions that would warrant immediate re-attention.
    Clear liquid diet.
    Acetaminophen at appropriate dose for age or weight.

Specific Measures. See specific diagnosis protocols.

Physician Consultation. For all children under 6 months and for any suspected of potential acute abdomen. Also consult when uncertain of working diagnosis or for therapeutic failure.

Referral.

Immediate Transfer. For acute abdomen to _____.

Follow-up Plan. Remind parents that patient should be rechecked in _____ days, immediately if worse.

	Initials	Date
* unless allergic, contraindicated, or pregnant/lactating	Physician ARNP	

Abdominal Pain (Non-Gynecologic and Non-Traumatic), Adults

EVALUATION/DIAGNOSTIC PROTOCOL

<u>Subjective</u>

History. Detailed description of pain beginning with characteristics and **location** at onset and subsequently. Detail aggravating and alleviating factors, radiating and accompanying symptomatology, previous similar symptomatology or abdominal surgery. Review past medical history. Any recent use of drugs (over-the-counter, prescription, illicit)? L.M.P.

<u>Objective</u>

Physical Examination. General appearance, vital signs, ENT, chest, abdomen, and rectal. (Pelvic exam is necessary in differentiating from gynecologic causes).

Lab. Stool guiac, stool obtained on rectal exam and UA(hold for C&S). Consider stool for ova and parasites, stool for enteric pathogen, or if **acute abdomen**, consider CBC, chemistry panel(including electrolytes and enzymes), serum amylase, chest x-ray with flat and upright abdominal series. Always do HCG in fertile women.

<u>Assessment</u>. Try to decide whether or not this is an acute abdomen. It is most common for pain to be the result of viral, bacterial, protozoal, gastroenteritis, or intestinal parasites. (See <u>Gastroenteritis in Adults</u>.) Consider medications and/or other ingestants. **Differential diagnosis** is multitudinous the more common causes of acute abdomen include (see <u>Peptic Ulcer Disease)</u>, gastroesophagitis, cholecystic disease, pancreatititis, diverticulitis, appendicitis, intestinal obstuction or ischemia, renal colic (see <u>Pyelonephritis</u> or <u>Nephrolitiasis</u>), aortic aneurysm, and causes which seem abdominal including myocardial ischemia and bibasilar intrathoracic processes. Gynecologic causes include P.I.D., ectopic pregnancy, ovarian cyst, and endometriosis. **Complications** depend on etiology.

<u>PLAN</u>/**MANAGEMENT PROTOCOL**

General Measures. Review with patient likely and suspected diagnosis and particular signs or symptoms of acute abdominal conditions that would warrant immediate re-attention. Clear liquid diet. Acetaminophen at appropriate dose for age or weight. Advise patient of the necessity of witholding strong analgesia until etiology is known.

Specific Measures. Depend entirely on the working differential diagnosis.

Physician Consultation for all suspected of potential acute abdomen. Also consult when uncertain of working diagnosis or for therapeutic failure.

Referral. Upon physician consultation.

Immediate Transfer for acute abdomen.

Follow-up Plan. Remind patient to be rechecked in _____ days, immediately if worse.

	Initials	Date
* unless allergic, contraindicated, or pregnant/lactating	Physician ARNP	

CHAPTER 3
OPHTHALMIC

Conjunctivitis

EVALUATION/DIAGNOSTIC PROTOCOL
Subjective
History. Course of symptoms. Question carefully about foreign bodies, irritants, and other infections. Do family, friends, co-workers, classmates have this also? Any history of Herpes I or II? Contact lens use?

Objective
Physical Examination. Complete eye exam. Acuity, lids, conjunctiva (fluorescein), cornea, pupils, retina, and EOM. In children, additionally perform complete ENT exam.

Lab. Consider gram stain and/or culture and sensitivity, though most often these are viral.

Assess severity. Be suspicious of Chlamydia, gonorrhea in newborns. Differential Diagnosis would include obstructed tear duct, herpes, iritis, abrasion, foreign body, as well as allergic reaction (pruritis predominate symptom), chemical irritant, upper respiratory tract infections including sinusitus. Complications are rare but include keratitis, corneal ulceration or scarring.

PLAN/MANAGEMENT PROTOCOL
General Measures. Explain to patient or parent that most commonly conjunctivitis is a viral infection sometimes just involving the conjunctiva and sometimes as part of a viral U.R.I. and a s such is self-limited. Good hygiene, frequent hand-washing, cold compressing.

Specific Measures.
Rx for antibiotic drops _____ *(MIS)
                              or
alternative drops_____ *(MIS)

                      or
Rx for antibiotic ointment_____ *(MIS)
                      or
alternative ointment _____ *(MIS).

Physician Consultation. Consider for severe discomfort, marked findings, infants under one month or as discussed below. Also consider if no improvement in _____ hours or if worsening.

Referral.

Immediate Referral. Suspected iritis, acute glaucoma, herpes, persistent foreign body, alkali injury.

Follow-up Plan. Recheck in _____ hours if not considerably improved, sooner if worse.

                                                    Initials   Date

* unless allergic, contraindicated,   Physician
or pregnant/lactating   ARNP

Hordeolum (Sty) & Chalazion

EVALUATION/DIAGNOSTIC PROTOCOL

<u>Subjective</u>
History. Symptoms and course.

<u>Objective</u>
Physical Examination. Complete eye exam; visual acuity, lids, conjunctiva, cornea, pupil, retina, EOMs.

Lab. Not necessary.

<u>Assess</u> severity. **Differential Diagnosis** is between hordeolum, chalazion, benign and malignant tumors. **Complications.** Periorbital cellulitis which can be life threatening.

<u>PLAN</u>/**MANAGEMENT PROTOCOL**
General Measures. Hot compress 15 minutes 3-4 times a day for adults and cooperative children. Emphasize good hand washing technique to prevent spread. No eye make-up. Remove contact lenses for _____ days after infection resolved.

Specific Measures.
Consider topical antibiotic Rx _____*(MIS)
                                                    or
alternative topical Rx _____*(MIS)

                                                    or
Oral antibiotic Rx _____*(MIS)
                                                    or
alternative oral Rx _____*(MIS).

Physician Consultation. Consider for fluctuant lesion, periorbital swelling, history of preceding trauma or severe pain if not resolved in 10 days, sooner if worsening.

Referral.

Immediate Transfer. If I and D indicated to ophthalmologist _____ or if periorbital cellulitis to _____.

Follow-up Plan. If not resolved in 3 days or sooner if worse.

	Initials	Date
* unless allergic, contraindicated,	Physician	
or pregnant/lactating	ARNP	

Corneal Abrasion & Foreign Body

EVALUATION/DIAGNOSTIC PROTOCOL
<u>Subjective</u>
History. Circumstances of injury. Course and severity of symptoms.

<u>Objective</u>
Physical Examination. Complete eye exam; visual acuity, lids, conjunctiva, cornea (stained with fluorescein instilling _____ anesthetic drop--option), pupils, retina, EOMs. Diagram location of abrasion.

Lab. Not necessary.

<u>Assess</u> to be certain no foreign body remains. **Complications** are secondary infection, corneal scarring, or those associated with penetrating foreign body (hyphema).

PLAN/MANAGEMENT PROTOCOL
General Measures. Emphasize to patient the need to keep patch secure.
  No contact lenses for _____ days after abrasion healed.

Specific Measures. Patch for 12-24 hours.
Consider instilling an antibiotic ointment and Rx _____*(MIS)
                                          or
alternative antibiotic ointment _____*(MIS).

Physician Consultation. For persistent superficial foreign body, severe pain or injury, or for abrasion not completely healed when second recheck performed at 48 hours.

Referral.

Immediate referral. To ophthalmologist for deep or penetrating foreign body or any metallic foreign body.

Follow-up Plan. Recheck in _____ hours and again in _____ hours if abrasion not completely healed. If resolved and patient without symptoms ask them to phone in.

	Initials	Date
* unless allergic, contraindicated, or pregnant/lactating	Physician	
	ARNP	

<u>Dacrocystitis & Obstructed Tear Ducts</u>
(<u>Lacrimal System Inflammation &</u>)

EVALUATION/DIAGNOSTIC PROTOCOL
<u>Subjective</u>
History. Onset and course of symptoms (tearing, discharge, swelling?).

<u>Objective</u>
Physical Examination. As thorough an eye exam as the infant allows and ENT exam.

Lab. Consider culture and sensitivities if recurrent.

<u>Assess</u> severity. **Differential Diagnosis.** Acute dacrocystitis, chronic tear duct obstruction, and the few rare systemic causes. **Complications.** Enlargement of the lacrimal gland.

<u>PLAN/MANAGEMENT PROTOCOL</u>
General Measures Explain where tears are made and that these drain into the the nose through a small adjacent opening. This usually represents a plumbing problem (an obstruction in the lacrimal passages due to epithelial remnants in the duct or membranous occlusion) which can be relieved by simple pressure on the tear sac that lies in the nose corner of each eye socket. Pressure should be applied gently, daily, with clean finger (nail cut short) several times a day.

Specific Measures
If infection is suspected consider topical antibiotic Rx _____*(MIS).

Physician Consultation.

Referral. To ophthamologist for any infant who has not responded to _____ weeks of therapy, preferably before age three to six months, so that the duct can be probed open without general anesthesia.

Immediate Transfer.

Follow-up Plan. In _____ weeks or as indicated.

	Initials	Date
* unless allergic, contraindicated, or pregnant/lactating	Physician ARNP	

Glaucoma

EVALUATION/DIAGNOSTIC PROTOCOL
Subjective
History. Onset and course of symptoms (to help distinguish between open-angle and angle-closure). Ask specifically about blurred or foggy vision with colored halos around lights, pain (follows trigeminal nerve pattern), nausea/vomiting. Medical history. Drug history. Family history of glaucoma?

Objective
Physical Examination. Vision test (Snellen). Complete eye exam. Open-angle: look for cupping or asymmetry of the optic disc or changes in visual fields. Closed angle: the eye is red and painful, the pupil may be unreactive to light, bradycardia, diaphoresis, signs of autonomic stimulation. If using dilating drops, you need to perform a penlight exam of the anterior chamber to insure it is normal and deep (especially in someone over 50).

Lab. Refer to _____ for evaluation of intraocular pressure by applanation tonometry unless available in your facility. Simple Schiotz tonometry can be inaccurate and has limited value, even in a screening setting.

Assess whether this is open-angle glaucoma or angle-closure glaucoma; both can cause blindness but acute angle closure is a serious ophthalmologic emergency! **Differential Diagnosis** is to determine whether this is primary open-angle, angle-closure, or glaucoma that is secondary to either another local cause or systemic disease. **Complications**. Blindness.

PLAN/MANAGEMENT PROTOCOL
General Measures. Explain to patient the importance of following through with the referral. Stress the importance of annual re-evaluation for anyone over forty, particularly if family history is positive for glaucoma. Discuss importance of compliance with medical regimen, teach possible side effects and reinforce need to continue treatment to avoid blindness.

Specific Measures. Rx usually prescribed by consulting ophthalmologist.

Physician Consultation. Whenever you suspect acute angle-closure glaucoma, this is an ophthalmologic emergency. Consider when suspecting open-angle, or if diagnoses is in doubt.

Referral. To _____ immediately if suspect acute angle-closure glaucoma or to _____ for a scheduled thorough ophthalmologic evaluation as appropriate for age.

Follow-Up Plan. Usually by ophthalmologist. Review during preventive care routine visits or if presenting symptoms lead you to question condition or medication side effects.

	Initials	Date
* unless allergic, contraindicated,	Physician	
or pregnant/lactating	ARNP	

Cataracts

EVALUATION/DIAGNOSTIC PROTOCOL
<u>Subjective</u>
History. Onset and course of symptoms. Any recent or remote history of trauma? Any underlying or predisposing conditions (diabetes)?

<u>Objective</u>
Physical Examination. Complete visual exam; acuity, lids, conjunctiva, sclera, cornea, pupils, lens (retina), EOM.

Lab. None.

<u>Assess</u> severity of opacification. **Differential Diagnosis** from glaucomatous changes. **Complications.** Visual impairment.

PLAN/MANAGEMENT PROTOCOL
General Measures. Discuss the need for regular opthalmalogic follow-up.

Specific Measures. Are instituted by opthalmologists.

Physician Consultation. If signs or symptoms of glaucoma. (See <u>Glaucoma</u>.)

Referral. Refer to ophthalmologist upon initial discovery and at recommended frequency thereafter.

Immediate Transfer. Not necessary.

Follow-up Plan. By ophthalmologist.

	Initials	Date
* unless allergic, contraindicated, or pregnant/lactating	Physician	
	ARNP	

CHAPTER 4
OTORHINOLARYNGOLOGIC

Inspissated Cerumen

EVALUATION/DIAGONSTIC PROTOCOL
__Subjective__
History. Course, review hygienic practices, past medical history, and family history.

__Objective__
Physical Examination. Complete ear exam.

Lab. Usually not necessary.

__Assess__ severity. **Differential Diagnosis** includes other exernal auditory canal masses including foreign bodies and neoplasms. **Complications** include otitis externa.

PLAN/MANAGEMENT PROTOCOL
General Measures.
Recommend use of OTC softening drops_____*(MIS).

Specific Measures. Remove cerumen either with cerumen spoon or by irrigation.

Consider topical antibiotic drops if any significant degree of external auditory canal epithelial trauma.

Physician Consultation. Consider if unable to easily remove cerumen or if untoward effect of your attempt. Also consider for diagnostic uncertainty.

Referral.

Follow-up Plan. Annually.

Acute Otitis Media, Infants and Children

EVALUATION/DIAGNOSTIC PROTOCOL
<u>Subjective</u>
History. Onset and course, other ENT symptoms, and other accompanying symptoms (feeding difficulty, frequent awakening, and occasional diarrhea). General medical history, past history, family history (allergies?). Any predisposing factors (smokers in the household, communal day care settings)?

<u>Objective</u>
Physical Examination. Vital signs, general appearance, complete ENT exam (w/ or w/o pneumatic otoscopy), neck, chest.

Lab. Usually not necessary, though tympanometry may be useful in quantifying resolution.

<u>Assess</u> severity, not only of appearance of the middle ear(s) but beyond that how this episode fits in the child's pattern, if any, of recurring infections and currently how ill is the patient. **Differential Diagnosis** is directed more at the possible infecting pathogen and association with invasive disease. **Complications** can be local, such as chronic serous effusion, perforation, mastoiditis or systemic, including bacteremia and meningitis.

PLAN/MANAGEMENT PROTOCOL
General Measures. Recommend age/weight appropriate dosing with acetaminophen for pain or fever. Explain to the parents the anatomy and physiology of the middle ear and how it is compromised by this infection and that this is a variable phenomenon. Discuss possible ways to limit these. Emphasize seriousness of this problem and the need for follow-up visits, in particular if recurrent.

   If tympanic membrane perforated, give detailed instructions about ear care (keeping water out of canals, gently removing and cleaning discharge and debris from canal opening). Provide <u>Middle Ear Infection</u> instruction sheet.

Specific Measures.
Initial oral antibiotic Rx _____*(MIS)
                                    or
alternative oral antibiotic Rx _____*(MIS).

If the child has a pattern of frequent refractory infections or there is a recent family/community history of resistant bacterial strains, then

Consider oral antibiotic _____*(MIS)
                                    or
as an alternative Rx _____*(MIS).

If perforation, consider additional topical Rx _____*(MIS).

Physician Consultation. If child is under _____ months or if severely ill. Consider for frequent, refractory or severe episodes or for more than _____ episodes in one year or as indicated.

Referral.

Immediate Transfer. May be necessary for the toxic/septic child.

Follow-up Plan. Recheck in _____ days or sooner if worse.

                                                    Initials   Date

* unless allergic, contraindicated,   Physician
or pregnant/lactating   ARNP

Serous Otitis Media, Infants and Children

EVALUATION/DIAGNOSTIC PROTOCOL

Subjective

History. Recent course, note ENT symptoms (hearing difficulties?). Any predisposing factors (bottle use, smokers in the household, communal day care settings, family history of allergies)? Immunization status?

Objective

Physical Examination. Vital signs, general appearance, complete ENT exam (w/ or w/o pneumatic otoscopy), neck, chest.

Lab. Usually not necessary, though tympanometry may be useful in quantifying resolution especially if not regularly performing pneumatic otoscopy.

Assess chronicity. **Differential Diagnosis** would include mechanical dysfunction, ("glue ear," eustachean dysfunction, etc.), allergic rhinitis, and possible infecting pathogen(s). **Complications** include re-infection, cholesteatoma, hearing impairment.

PLAN/MANAGEMENT PROTOCOL

General Measures. Explain to the parents the anatomy and physiology of the middle ear and how it is compromised by this infection. Discuss possible ways to limit these. Discuss bottle propping, advantage of continued nursing, isolating the child from excessive exposure to sick kids, allergy-proofing the environment [see Allergy-Proofing the Bedroom], in particular providing smoke-free setting).

Emphasize seriousness of this problem, the need for follow-up visits, and giving prescriptions as prescribed.

Specific Measures.
Consider oral antibiotic Rx _____*(MIS)

or

alternative, oral antibiotic _____*(MIS) for a prolonged course of treatment _____ weeks. Note: Caution should be exercised in choice of antibiotics.

Consider pneumococcal vaccine.

Physician Consultation. Consider if child is under _____ months or if severely ill. Consider if refractory, for more than _____ episodes in one year or as indicated. Discuss myringotomy with placement of tympanostomy tubes and possibility of adenoidectomy.

Referral.

Immediate Transfer. May be necessary for the toxic/septic child.

Follow-up Plan. Recheck in _____ days/weeks.

Initials   Date

* unless allergic, contraindicated,   Physician
or pregnant/lactating   ARNP

Acute Otitis Media, Adults

EVALUATION/DIAGNOSTIC PROTOCOL
Subjective
History. General history course and ENT symptoms, family exposure or occupational exposure to sick children. Any predisposing factors (smoking or smokers in the household, personal or family history of allergies)?

Objective
Physical Examination. Vital signs, general appearance, complete ENT exam (w/ or w/o pneumatic otoscopy), neck, chest.

Lab. Usually not necessary, though tympanometry may be useful in quantifying resolution.

Assess severity. **Differential Diagnosis** is directed more at the possible infecting pathogen and association with invasive disease. **Complications** can be local, such as chronic serous effusion, perforation, mastoiditis or systemic infection.

PLAN/MANAGEMENT PROTOCOL
General Measures.
Recommend appropriate nonnarcotic analgesic _____*(MIS).
Consider narcotic analgesic _____*(MIS).

Specific Measures.
Initial oral antibiotic Rx _____*(MIS)
or
alternative antibiotic Rx _____*(MIS).

If exposure to sick children, consider alternative oral antibiotics.
Rx _____*(MIS)
or
Rx _____*(MIS).

If perforation, consider additional topical Rx _____*(MIS).

Physician Consultation. Consider for severe infections or development of complications.

Referral.

Follow-up Plan. Recheck in _____ days/weeks if indicated.

Initials   Date

* unless allergic, contraindicated,   Physician
or pregnant/lactating   ARNP

Otitis Externa

EVALUATION/DIAGNOSTIC PROTOCOL
Subjective
History. Symptoms and course (consider foreign body and/or trauma). Are there predisposing factors or underlying conditions (diabetes).

Objective
Physical Examination. Complete ear exam. Consider complete ENT exam.

Lab. Usually not necessary.

Assessment severity and etiology (in addition to the more common fungal and bacterial causes consider Herpes simplex). **Differential Diagnosis** includes otitis media with perforation, injury, or manifestations of the chronic and acute dermatitidies including atopic, contact, seborrheic, and psoriasis. **Complications** include cellulitis and mastoiditis either of which can be life-threatening in the diabetic.

PLAN/MANAGEMENT PROTOCOL
General Measures. In other words, keep ear dry for _____ days (no swimming and careful bathing). Consider age appropriate OTC oral analgesic. When fully recovered to prevent future infections after swimming fill external auditory canal with a solution of 1/2 white vinegar and 1/2 rubbing alcohol or similar OTC product _____. (Remind the patient not to drain the solution into the eyes). Remind patients to avoid manipulating ear canals. This includes not using cotton swabs. Provide Swimmer's Ear Infection instruction sheet.

Special Measures. Manually remove as much debris as possible.

Consider placing a _____ wick for 24 hours. (Instruct patient in removal).

Moisten wick with topical Rx _____.

Prescribe topical Rx _____ *(MIS)
                                    and/or
alternative topical _____ *(MIS).

Consider oral antibiotic _____ *(MIS).

Physician Consultation. Consider for severe infection, severe pain, or if persistent or recurring.

Referral.

Immediate Referral. For severe cellulitis in a diabetic.

Follow-up. In _____ day(s) or sooner, depending upon severity.

                                                    Initials   Date
* unless allergic, contraindicated,   Physician
or pregnant/lactating   ARNP

Allergic Rhinitis, Children

EVALUATION/DIAGNOSTIC PROTOCOL
Subjective.
History. Child's symptoms and variations (seasonal and/or circumstantial) as well as aggravating (smokers or pets in the home) and alleviating factors. Any family history of allergies, asthma, or eczema/atopy?

Objective
Physical Examination. General appearance, eyes, ears, nose and throat, lungs, and skin.

Lab. Testing usually not necessary. If history not definitive, consider _____.

Assess severity. **Differential Diagnosis** would include URI, nasal foreign body obstruction, sinus infection. **Complications**. Serous otitis media, sinusitis, and nasal polyps.

PLAN/MANAGEMENT PROTOCOL
General Measures. Remind parent that allergies can usually be controlled but not cured. Over-the-counter medication should be avoided. Avoid tobacco smoke and other air pollutants. Consider keeping pets out of the house and car. In particular, allergy-proof the bedroom (see Allergy-Proofing the Bedroom). Encourage plenty of sleep and good nutrition.

Specific Measures.
Oral antihistamine Rx _____*(MIS)
                                         or
alternative antihistamine Rx _____*(MIS)
(or others as indicated by patient's history and working through other antihistamine families not previously used).
                                         or
Oral antihistamine/decongestant Rx _____*(MIS)
                                         or
alternative antihistamine/decongestant Rx _____*(MIS).
                                         or
Topical nasal therapy Rx _____*(MIS).

Physician Consultation. If uncertain of the diagnosis or if intolerant or refractory to therapeutic trial.

Referral.

Follow-up Plan. Recheck in _____ week(s)/month(s) or as indicated.

	Initials	Date
* unless allergic, contraindicated,	Physician	
or pregnant/lactating	ARNP	

Allergic Rhinitis, Adults

EVALUATION/DIAGNOSTIC PROTOCOL
Subjective.
History. Personal symptoms and variations (seasonal and/or circumstantial) as well as aggravating and alleviating factors. Any family history of allergies, asthma, or eczema/atopy. Past medical history. Medication useage?   Last menstrual period.

Objective
Physical Examination. General appearance, eyes, ears, nose and throat, lungs.

Lab. Testing usually not necessary. If history not definitive, consider
_____.

Assess severity. **Differential Diagnosis** includes URI, sinus infection.
Complications. Sinusitis.

PLAN/MANAGEMENT PROTOCOL
General Measures. Remind patient that allergies can usually be controlled but not cured. Prescription medication should be taken as prescribed. Over-the-counter medication should be avoided. Avoid tobacco smoke and other air pollutants. Consider keeping pets out of the house and car. In particular, allergy-proof the bedroom (see Allergy-Proofing the Bedroom). Encourage plenty of sleep and good nutrition.

Specific Measures.
Oral antihistamine Rx _____*(MIS)
                                    or
alternative antihistamine Rx _____*(MIS)
(or others as indicated by patient's history and working through other antihistamine families not previously used).

                                    or
Oral antihistamine/decongestant Rx _____*(MIS)
                                    or
alternative antihistamine/decongestant Rx _____*(MIS).

                                    or
Topical nasal therapy Rx _____*(MIS)
                                    or
alternative topical Rx _____*(MIS).

Physician Consultation. If intolerant or refractory to therapeutic trial.

Referral.

Follow-up Plan. Recheck in _____ week(s)/month(s) or as indicated.

                                                    Initials   Date
* unless allergic, contraindicated,   Physician
or pregnant/lactating   ARNP

Upper Respiratory Tract Infection, Children

EVALUATION/DIAGNOSTIC PROTOCOL

<u>Subjective</u>

History. Onset and course, any ENT symptoms, any other accompanying symptoms (feeding difficulty, frequent awakening, and occasional diarrhea)? General medical history, past history, family history (allergies?). Any predisposing factors (smokers in the household, communal day care settings)?

<u>Objective</u>.

Physical Examination. General appearance, vital signs, ENT, neck, chest.

Lab. None needed.

Assess severity. **Differential Diagnosis**. Sinusitis, allergic rhinitis. **Complications**. Otitis media, sinusitis.

<u>PLAN</u>/MANAGEMENT PROTOCOL

General Measures. Encourage rest, plenty of fluids, and well-balanced diet. For young infants consider gentle suction with rubber bulb aspirator. In general children do not benefit from oral decongestants. Provide the <u>Common Cold</u> instruction sheet.

    Consider salt water (saline) nose drops for infants, which should be made fresh daily by adding 1/2 teaspoon of table salt to 8 ounces of water. Then put 2-4 drops in each nostril just prior to feeding the infant and suck the drops and moistened mucus out with a rubber bulb aspirator (or use similar OTC preparation).

Specific Measures. There is no specific therapy for colds. There is symptomatic modification, acetaminophen.

Consider oral Rx _____ *(MIS).

Physician Consultation. All infants under _____ months of age.

Referral.

Follow-up Plan. In _____ day(s) if not improved, sooner if worsening symptoms or signs indicative of secondary bacterial infection.

                                                             Initials   Date

* unless allergic, contraindicated,   Physician
or pregnant/lactating   ARNP

Upper Respiratory Tract Infection, Adults

EVALUATION/DIAGNOSTIC PROTOCOL

Subjective

History. General history course and ENT symptoms, family exposure or exposure to others sick. Any predisposing factors (smoking or smokers in the household, personal or family history of allergies)?

Objective

Physical Examination. General appearance, vital signs, ENT, neck, chest.

Lab. None needed.

Assess severity. **Differential Diagnosis**. Sinusitis, allergic rhinitis. **Complications**. Sinusitis.

PLAN/MANAGEMENT PROTOCOL

General Measures. Encourage rest, plenty of fluids, and well-balanced diet.

Specific Measures. There is no specific therapy for colds. There is symptomatic modification, acetaminophen (or aspirin in adults who do not have allergic rhinitis or epistaxis).

Adults may benefit from decongestants, topical _____ *(MIS).

Oral Rx _____ *(MIS).

Physician Consultation. Usually not necessary.

Referral. Usually not necessary.

Follow-up Plan. In _____ day(s) if not improved, sooner if worsening symptoms or signs indicative of secondary bacterial infection.

		Initials	Date
* unless allergic, contraindicated, or pregnant/lactating	Physician ARNP		

Sinusitis, Children

EVALUATION/DIAGNOSTIC PROTOCOL

<u>Subjective</u>

History. Onset and course of symptoms which may be nonspecific (fever, malaise, headache) or specific (focal pain, nocturnal cough, and hallitosis). Previous history. Predisposing factors (smoker in the house) or underlying conditions.

<u>Objective</u>

Physical Examination. General appearance, vital signs, ENT (consider trans-illumination), neck, chest.

Lab. Consider sinus culture obtained indirectly (eye, nasal, or pharyngeal swab) or directly (visualizing sinal drainage or with endoscope). Consider sinus x-rays (CT or MRI, depending upon severity or chronicity).

<u>Assess</u> severity and contribution of obstructive phenomenon. **Differential Diagnosis.** Consider foreign body. **Complications** are bacteremia and meningitis as well as periorbital cellulitis and osteomyelitis.

<u>PLAN/MANAGEMENT PROTOCOL</u>

General Measures. Consider cool mist humidifier. Encourage increased fluid intake. For pain or fever, acetaminophen in appropriate dosages for weight or age.

Specific Measures.
Antibiotic Rx _____*(MIS)
                                         or
alternative antibiotic Rx _____*(MIS).

                                        and

Oral decongestant OTC/Rx _____*(MIS)
                                         or
alternative decongestant OTC/Rx _____*(MIS).

Physician Consultation. Consider depending upon severity, persistence, or recurrence. Consider more immediately for suspected complications.

Referral.

Immediate Transfer. May be necessary for toxic/septic child.

Follow-up Plan. Recheck in _____ days if not improved, sooner if worse.

		Initials	Date
* unless allergic, contraindicated,	Physician		
or pregnant/lactating	ARNP		

Sinusitis, Adults

EVALUATION/DIAGNOSTIC PROTOCOL
Subjective
History. Onset and course of symptoms. Any predisposing factors (smoking or smokers at home or in the workplace) or underlying conditions (allergic rhiniitis)?

Objective
Physical Examination. General appearance, vital signs, ENT, neck, chest.

Lab. Consider sinus x-rays. Consider nasal culture.

Assess severity and contribution of obstructive phenomenon. **Differential Diagnosis** includes intranasal or intrasinal mass when patient has recurring or refractory symptoms. These must be differentiated from various types of headaches and the more significant causes: periorbital cellulits, cavernous sinus thrombosis and intra-cranial neoplasm. **Complications.** Periorbital cellulitis, bacteremia, osteomyelitis and meningitis.

PLAN/MANAGEMENT PROTOCOL
General Measures. A vaporizer (if no children in the house to knock it over) otherwise a cool mist humidifier or hot compresses may be helpful. Encourage increased fluid intake. For pain or fever, acetaminophen, aspirin, or ibuprofen.

Specific Measures.
Antibiotic Rx _____*(MIS)
                                     or
alternative antibiotic Rx _____*(MIS).

                                     and

Oral decongestant OTC/Rx _____*(MIS)
                                     or
alternative decongestant OTC/Rx _____*(MIS).

Physician Consultation. Depending upon severity, persistence, or recurrence. Consider more immediately for suspected complications.

Referral.

Immediate Transfer. For more serious sequellae.

Follow-up Plan. Recheck in _____ days if not improved, sooner if worse.

	Initials	Date
* unless allergic, contraindicated,	Physician	
or pregnant/lactating	ARNP	

Epistaxis

EVALUATION/DIAGNOSTIC PROTOCOL
Subjective

History. Obtain immediate past history of circumstances surrounding the onset of bleeding and the course. Is there accompanying symptomatology (orthostasis), previous history of epistaxis? Current medications, both prescription and nonprescription.

Objective

Physical Examination. General appearance, vital signs, ENT exam with gentle examination of the nose with attention directed at Kiesselbach's plexus on the lower nasal septal mucosa.

Lab if history suggestive consider testing for clotting disorders.

Assessment is directed at whether the bleeding is anterior or posterior. Differential diagnosis. Consider foreign body in children. Consider malignancy in adults. Complications relate to amount of bleeding.

PLAN/MANAGEMENT PROTOCOL
General Measures. Remind patient or parents that nosebleeds occur most commonly as a result of injury, such as from picking the nose or from trauma. This is also more common with colds when the lining of the nose is irritated from the infection and during the winter when excessive drying of the inner surface of the nose causes bleeding

Sit the patient up and lean him/her forward so they are not swallowing blood. Pinch the nose between thumb and forefinger for five minutes. Instruct the patient to breathe through the mouth. An ice pack may be placed over the bridge of the nose to diminish blood flow.

If bleeding stops, instruct the parents or patient to treat the nose gently, avoiding blowing or rubbing to excess. The next day, begin to lubricate inside the nostrils with over-the-counter antibiotic ointment.

Specific Measures. Specific measures involving packing or cauterizing usually instituted by the physician.

Physician Consultation. For any patient exhibiting orthostasis or hypotension, or for bleeding not controlled by _____ minutes of ice pack and compression.

Immediate Referral. For evidence of severe bleeding or suspected posterior bleed to _____.

Follow-up Plan. As needed.

	Initials	Date
* unless allergic, contraindicated, or pregnant/lactating	Physician ARNP	

Pharyngitis and Tonsillitis

EVALUATION/DIAGNOSTIC PROTOCOL

Subjective

History. Onset and course of symptoms. Predisposing factors or underlying conditions. General medical history.

Objective

Physical Examination. General appearance, vital signs, ENT, neck for nodes, liver and spleen.

Lab. Strep culture or rapid strep test, consider CBC and mono.

Assess severity and degree of tonsillar enlargement. **Differential Diagnosis.** Consider viral pharyngitis, mycoplasma, aphthous stomatitis, mononucleosis, bacterial tonsillitis. **Complications.** Peritonsillar abscess, rheumatic fever is a complication of strep.

PLAN/MANAGEMENT PROTOCOL

General Measures. For young children and infants, cool soothing liquids may be helpful. For older children or adults, consider warm saline gargles.

For pain, acetaminophen for children or adults (aspirin for adults only). Doses need to be appropriate for weight and/or age. For particular painful throats or marked tonsillitis with dysphagia, encourage extra nutritious and non-irritating liquids such as milk shakes.

Specific Measures.

For adults with strep pharyngitis, give oral Rx _____*(MIS).

For children with strep pharyngitis, give oral Rx _____*(MIS).

or

as an alternative, consider I.M. benzathine penicillin.

For viral, no treatment necessary.

Physician Consultation. Consider for severe or prolonged symptoms, peritonsilar abscess, severe cervical lymphadenitis.

Referral.

Immediate Transfer. May be necessary for peritonsillar abscess.

Follow-up Plan. As needed or if persistent symptoms after _____ days or sooner if worsening.

	Initials	Date
* unless allergic, contraindicated, or pregnant/lactating	Physician	
	ARNP	

Aphthous Stomatitis/Aphthous Ulcers

EVALUATION/DIAGNOSTIC PROTOCOL

<u>Subjective</u>

History. Onset and course of symptoms. Prior history? Preceding illness? Any predisposing factors or underlying conditions?

<u>Objective</u>.

Physical Examination. For children, vital signs, general appearance, complete ENT exam, and neck exam. For adults, thorough examination of the mouth.

Lab. Usually none.

<u>Assessment</u>. Multiple lesions may represent a true primary stomatitis in children. A limited number of ulcers is usually a recurrance. **Differential Diagnosis** for stomatitis includes; Herpes simplex, herpangina, Behcet's syndrome and for only a few lesions again consider herpes. **Complications** in the young child relate to limited oral intake because of pain.

<u>PLAN/MANAGEMENT PROTOCOL</u>

General Measures. Remind patients and parents that most sores heal within 5-10 days. Avoid citrus fruits and juices and spicy foods. Encourage plenty of cool, soothing liquids, particularly milkshakes and milk. Yogurt seems particularly helpful. Consider analgesia with acetaminophen in appropriate dose for weight or age.

Specific Measures. Consider recommending oral preparations containing hydrogen peroxide. Consider treatment with silver nitrate application. Consider other oral mucosal topicals _____*(MIS).

Physician Consultation. Consider for severely ill infants and young children who are not feeding properly, inordinate recurrences, or diagnostic uncertainty.

Referral. Usually not necessary.

Follow-up Plan. If sores persist beyond one week.

	Initials	Date
* unless allergic, contraindicated, or pregnant/lactating	Physician ARNP	

Oral Candidiasis

EVALUATION/DIAGNOSTIC PROTOCOL
Subjective
History. Onset and course of symptoms. Predisposing factors (in particular any recent antibiotic use) or underlying conditions? Known exposure?

Objective
Physical Examination. General, ENT, and on infants complete exam.

Lab. Consider KOH prep. Consider FBS and/or HIV testing in adults with severe infection or recurrences.

Assess severity. **Differential Diagnosis.** Aphthous ulcers, herpes and other gingival infections and conditions. **Complications** in infants difficulty feeding leading to volume depletion.

PLAN/MANAGEMENT PROTOCOL
General Measures. For infants, wash all baby's nipples, pacifiers, utensils. Practice good hand-washing technique. Instruct parents in application and administration of oral antifungal. For infants, a drop should be placed in a small cup, a swab dipped into the medicine, applied to patches in the baby's mouth. Repeat until the entire dose has been swallowed. Older children can be directed to swish the medicine around the mouth before swallowing. Nursing mother may need nipple and areola treatment.

Specific Measures.
For infants and children, Rx _____*(MIS).

For adults, oral Rx _____*(MIS).

Physician Consultation. Consider for persistent or recurrent infection.

Referral. Not usually necessary.

Follow-up Plan. Recheck in _____ days if not considerably improved, sooner if worse.

	Initials	Date
* unless allergic, contraindicated,	Physician	
or pregnant/lactating	ARNP	

CHAPTER 5
RESPIRATORY

Croup/Laryngotracheobronchitis

EVALUATION/DIAGNOSTIC PROTOCOL
Subjective
History. Determine the course and onset of symptoms, attempting to distinguish this from epiglottitis (sudden onset, rapid progression, high fever, drooling). What home measures have been tried?

Objective
Physical Examination. General appearance, vital signs, ENT exam, unless there is a high index of suspicion of epiglottitis (lethargic-toxic, or agitated, respiratory distress as evidenced by marked stridor and drooling), a life-threatening emergency.

Lab. None, if obviously LTB.

Assess the likelihood that you are dealing with a true viral croup and are not dealing with epiglottitis. (Often, the croup patient will improve on the way to the office because of the micro climate change.) **Differential diagnosis** includes epiglottitis, which, again, is a life-threatening, foreign body aspiration, also life-threatening, and laryngomalacia. **Complications**. Airway obstruction.

PLAN/MANAGEMENT PROTOCOL
General Measures. Explain to the parent that croup is a viral infection affecting the airway, but is usually without serious complications. Emphasize the need for parents to remain calm. The best treatment is to breathe moist air. This can be done by steaming up the bathroom and sitting calmly with the child for 15-30 minutes breathing the steam or by using a cool mist humidifier in the bedroom. Sometimes even a walk outside helps. Encourage plenty of fluids.
   If there is fever, treat with appropriate dose for age/weight of acetaminophen.

Specific Measures.
Do/Don't consider an mild cough suppressant _____*(MIS)

Physician Consultation. If suspected epiglottitis, refer **immediately**. Similarly, consult for any toxic child or with significant degree of respiratory distress.

Immediate Transfer. For suspected epiglottitis.

Follow-up Plan. If improvement not noticed with the usual croup measures, there is breathing difficulty, vomiting, gagging, choking, muffled voice, considerable drooling or general worsening in the appearance of the child, then the parent should be instructed to call the doctor **immediately**. Otherwise follow-up in _____ days.

	Initials	Date
Physician		
ARNP		

*unless allergic, contraindicated, or pregnant/lactating

Influenza (Children and Adults)

EVALUATION/DIAGNOSTIC PROTOCOL
<u>Subjective</u>
History. Onset and course of symptoms. Remember, this is a specific respiratory illness which should be occurring in the setting that others in the community are affected by the illness. Any predisposing factors or underlying conditions?

<u>Objective</u>
Physical Examination. General, vital signs, ENT, respiratory.

Lab. Often not necessary. Consider <u>CBC</u>, <u>chest x-ray</u>.

<u>Assess</u> severity, in particular as regards degree of respiratory distress.
Differential Diagnosis. Pneumonia, other viral respiratory syndromes and mycoplasm.
Complications. Respiratory distress or secondary pneumonia.

PLAN/MANAGEMENT PROTOCOL
General Measures. Reassure the patient that influenza is self-limiting and resolves quicker with rest. Keep the patient home from school and or work. Increased rest should be emphasized to the patient in an absolute unequivocal way. Tub baths will help with myalgias. Increase hydration. Symptomatic modification can be achieved with acetaminophen for children or adults (aspirin or ibuprofen for adults only). Doses need to be appropriate for weight and/or age.

Specific Measures.   FOR ADULTS
Early in the course consider Rx for amantadine _____*(MIS).

                                                   FOR CHILDREN
Early in the course consider Rx for amantadine _____*(MIS).

Physician Consultation. Depending upon severity and degree of respiratory distress.

Referral.

Immediate Transfer. For severe respiratory distress to _____.

Follow-up Plan. Recheck in _____ days if not considerably improved, sooner if worse.

	Initials	Date
*unless allergic, contraindicated, or pregnant/lactating	Physician ARNP	

Bronchiolitis

EVALUATION/DIAGNOSTIC PROTOCOL
Subjective
History. General and respiratory history. (Incidence most common under age 2, peaking at 6 months of age, most often during the winter.)

Objective
Physical Examination. General appearance, vital signs, ENT, chest (intercostal and subcostal retractions, widespread fine rales, prolonged expiratory phase, wheezing [be alarmed if breath sounds nearly inaudible]), cardiovascular, and abdomen.

Lab. Consider chest x-ray, CBC.

Assess degree of respiratory distress. **Differential Diagnosis** is asthma, LTB, pneumonia, pertussis, and foreign body aspiration. **Complications.** Severe respiratory distress with hypoxia, dehydration, and exhaustion.

PLAN/MANAGEMENT PROTOCOL
General Measures. Explain to parents the nature of this viral infection, which affects the small airway and causes the child to have difficulty breathing. Explain additionally that infants with significant respiratory distress require hospitalization and those with RSV can be treated with a relatively new medication.

Specific Measures. Are employed only in those infants with severe respiratory distress and in the hospital setting.

Physician Consultation. The authors recommend in most settings.

Referral.

Immediate Transfer. After consultation for significant respiratory distress.

Follow-up Plan. At the least consider daily phone follow-up. Otherwise recheck in _____ day(s).

Initials   Date

*unless allergic, contraindicated,   Physician
or pregnant/lactating   ARNP

Acute Bronchitis, Children

EVALUATION/DIAGNOSTIC PROTOCOL
Subjective
History. Onset and course of symptoms (could foreign body aspiration have occurred?). General and respiratory history. Any predisposing factors (smoking or smokers in the household, exposure to other inhalants, personal or family history of allergies) or underlying conditions? Medication usage?

Objective
Physical Examination. General, vital signs, ENT and chest.

Lab. This is mainly a clinical diagnosis. In some circumstances consider chest x-ray.

Assess severity and the possibility of bronchospasm. **Differential Diagnosis** includes asthma, bronchiolitis, foreign body aspiration, pneumonia (mycoplasma). **Complications.** Pneumonia and hypoxia.

PLAN/MANAGEMENT PROTOCOL
General Measures. Rest and plenty of fluids are the mainstay of therapy. Emphasize avoidance of passive smoking and other inhalants. Acetaminophen for children in doses appropriate to weight or age. Consider cool mist humidifier.
   Explain to patients or parents coughing is the way the lungs rid themselves of thick infected mucus. Cough suppressants should not be used except to allow sleep or performance of necessary activities. It may be helpful to use a simple lozenge or just a sucking candy to soothe the throat, if age appropriate. Similarly, caffeine containing beverages such as tea may be helpful because of their bronchodilator properties.

Specific Measures
For children give antibiotic Rx _____ *(MIS)
                                                  or
alternative Rx _____ *(MIS).
Consider appropriate bronchodilator therapy (see Asthma).
Consider cough suppressant Rx _____ *(MIS)
for use in the evenings only.

Physician Consultation. For toxic children or children with severe coughing or severe respiratory distress or suspected foreign body aspiration. Similarly, consult for persistent recurring symptomatology, as in asthmatics on bronchodilator therapy.

Referral.

Immediate Transfer. For severe respiratory distress or suspected foreign body.

Follow-up Plan. Recheck in _____ days if not improved, sooner if worse.

	Initials	Date
*unless allergic, contraindicated,	Physician	
or pregnant/lactating	ARNP	

Acute Bronchitis, Adults

EVALUATION/DIAGNOSTIC PROTOCOL
Subjective
History. Onset and course of symptoms. General and respiratory history. Any predisposing factors (smoking or smokers in the household, exposure to other inhalants, personal or family history of allergies) or underlying conditions? Medication usage?

Objective
Physical Examination. General, vital signs, ENT in chest.

Lab. This is mainly a clinical diagnosis. In some circumstances consider chest x-ray.

Assess severity and the possibility of bronchospasm, and chemical-induced or inhalant hypersensitivity. Similarly, evaluate for possible etiologic agents (viral, mycoplasma, bacterial, fungal). **Differential Diagnosis**. Asthma, pneumonia, pulmonary emboli. **Complications**. Pneumonia and hypoxia.

PLAN/MANAGEMENT PROTOCOL
General Measures. Rest and plenty of fluids are the mainstay of therapy. Emphasize avoiding smoking (either active or passive). Acetaminophen or aspirin. Consider cool mist humidifier.

Explain to patients coughing is the way the lungs rid themselves of thick infected mucus. Cough suppressants should not be used except to allow sleep or performance of necessary activities. It may be helpful to use a simple lozenge or just a sucking candy to soothe the throat. Similarly, caffeine containing beverages such as tea may be helpful because of their bronchodilator properties.

Specific Measures
For adults give antibiotic Rx _____ *(MIS)
or
alternative antibiotic _____ *(MIS).

Consider appropriate bronchodilator therapy (see Asthma).
Consider cough suppressant Rx _____ *(MIS)
for use in the evenings.

Physician Consultation. For adults with severe coughing or severe respiratory distress. Similarly, consult for persistent recurring symptomatology.

Referral. At the discretion of physician.

Immediate Transfer. For severe respiratory distress.

Follow-up Plan. Recheck in _____ days if not improved, sooner if worse.

	Initials	Date
*unless allergic, contraindicated, or pregnant/lactating	Physician ARNP	

Pneumonia, Children

EVALUATION/DIAGNOSTIC PROTOCOL
Subjective
History. Onset and course of symptoms (description of cough, duration of fever and/or chills, description of sputum). General and respiratory history, prediposing factors (smoker or smokers in the household, communal day care centers), or underlying conditions. Medications?

Objective
Physical Examination. General appearance (signs of respiratory distress), vital signs, ENT, chest (fine rales may be difficult to appreciate in small children or those with volume depletion), abdomen.

Lab. Consider CBC, chest x-ray, sputum smear, culture and sensitivity.

Assess severity by clinical indications of respiratory distress or by radiographic findings. Similarly, evaluate for possible etiologic agents in order to treat appropriately. **Differential Diagnosis** includes asthma, bronchiolitis, foreign body aspiration. **Complications** include dehydration, hypoxia, respiratory failure, and lung abscess.

PLAN/MANAGEMENT PROTOCOL
General Measures. Emphasize rest and plenty of fluids. Consider instructing family members in chest percussion and postural drainage. Some symptomatic relief can be obtained from acetaminophen in appropriate doses for weight. Place special emphasis on signs or symptoms of worsening that would require immediate attention.

Specific Measures.
Prescribe antibiotic _____ *(MIS)
                                        or
alternative antibiotic _____ *(MIS).

Physician Consultation. On all infants with pneumonia. Similarly, consult on all children with appearance other than that of mild infection or suspected underlying pathology.

Referral.

Immediate Transfer. May be necessary for the toxic/septic child.

Follow-up Plan. In _____ day(s) or sooner. Consider going to daily re-examination of infants and young children until there is clinical improvement.

	Initials	Date
*unless allergic, contraindicated, or pregnant/lactating	Physician ARNP	

Pneumonia, Adults

EVALUATION/DIAGNOSTIC PROTOCOL

Subjective

History. General and respiratory history, focused on recent circumstances, onset of symptoms, course of cough, duration of fever and/or chills, description of sputum, and whether there is a personal history of smoking or exposure to other inhalants. Is there a personal history of underlying or predisposing conditions? When was last menstrual period? Are there allergies to medications?

Objective

Physical Examination. General appearance (signs of respiratory distress), vital signs, ENT, and chest (fine rales).

Lab. Consider CBC, chest x-ray, sputum smear, culture and sensitivity.

Assess severity by clinical indications of respiratory distress or radiographic findings. Similarly, evaluate for possible etiologic agents (viral, mycoplasm, bacterial, most commonly pneumoccocal, fungal, or other). **Differential Diagnosis** includes bronchitis with bronchospasm. Consider evaluation for predisposing conditions. Remember, pneumonia is still a leading cause of death amongst the elderly. **Complications** include dehydration, hypoxia, respiratory failure, and/or lung abscess.

PLAN/MANAGEMENT PROTOCOL

General Measures. Emphasize rest and plenty of fluids. Consider instructing family members in chest percussion and postural drainage. Some symptomatic relief can be obtained from acetaminophen or aspirin. Place special emphasis on signs or symptoms of worsening that would require immediate follow-up.

Consider expectorant _____*(MIS).

Consider cough suppressant _____*(MIS).

Specific Measures.

Prescribe antibiotic with _____*(MIS)

or

as an alternative antibiotic _____*(MIS).

Physician Consultation. For other than obviously mild pneumonia, in the elderly. For any patient with complex health history or compromised immunity. For severe pneumonia or suspected unusual etiology, or for unusual radiographic appearance. For moderate to severe respiratory distress. Failure to respond to therapy or for sudden worsening are reasons for consulting or reconsulting.

Referral.

Immediate Transfer. If obvious toxicity or respiratory distress.

Follow-up Plan. In _____ day(s) or sooner as discussed above.

	Initials	Date
*unless allergic, contraindicated, or pregnant/lactating	Physician ARNP	

Chronic Bronchitis, Adults

EVALUATION/DIAGNOSTIC PROTOCOL

<u>Subjective</u>

History. General and respiratory (course of symptoms). Detailed smoking history. Occupational history. Family history.

<u>Objective</u>

Physical Examination. General appearance, vital signs, ENT, chest.

Lab. Consider CBC, Tb test, chest x-ray, spirometry or pulmonary function studies.

<u>Assess</u> severity of compromise of pulmonary function. It may be useful to try to classify the patient as predominantly emphysemic ("pink puffer") or as predominantly bronchitic ("blue bloater"). **Differential Diagnosis** includes pneumonia, acute bronchitis, tuberculosis, asthma, and congestive heart failure. Remember: in non-smoking families alpha-1 antitrypsin deficiency. **Complications** include pneumonia, hypoxia, respiratory failure, cor pulmonale, and cardiac arrhythmias.

<u>PLAN/MANAGEMENT PROTOCOL</u>

General Measures. Patient teaching about preventing complications and learning to live with C.O.P.D. Consider community support or education group. **Emphasize avoiding smoking** (either active or passive). Consider cool mist humidifier or vaporizer. Explain to patients coughing is the way the lungs rid themselves of thick infected mucus. Cough suppressants should not be used except to allow sleep or performance of necessary activities. It may be helpful to use a simple lozenge or just suck candy to soothe the throat. Similarly, caffeine containing beverages such as tea may be helpful because of their bronchodilator properties. Advise yearly influenza vaccine and one time pneumoccal vaccine.

Specific Measures. Consider SHORT (_____ days) or LONG (_____ weeks) COURSE antibiotic Rx _____*(MIS)

or

_____*(MIS).

If bronchospasm, consider bronchodilator therapy with inhalant Rx _____ or _____*(MIS)

and/or

Oral bronchodilator Rx _____*(MIS).

Physician Consultation. If diagnostic uncertainty. Consider urgently for signs of respiratory distress or worsening persistent symptomotology. Consider for persistent symptomatology for patient already on long course or before prescribing long course.

Referral.

Immediate Transfer.

Follow-up Plan. Individualized depending on severity of respiratory difficulty. and remind the patient to return whenever worsening.

	Initials	Date
*unless allergic, contraindicated,	Physician	
or pregnant/lactating	ARNP	

Acute Asthma (Children)

EVALUATION/DIAGNOSTIC PROTOCOL
Subjective
History. General and respiratory history. Emphasis on history of allergic disorders, both personal and familial. Try to ascertain precipitating factor (infection the most common [occult sinusitis most difficult to diagnose], but also consider allergy, environmental change, exercise). It is important to assess family history of allergic disorders. Remember that more than 10% of asthmatics may never wheeze but instead have a history of coughing and have been labeled as having recurring acute bronchitis. Obtain meticulous history of medications used in the past 36 hours, including amounts and times taken.

Objective
Physical Examination. General appearance, vital signs, ENT, chest, cardiac exam.

Lab. Laboratory tests may not be necessary. For infection, consider chest x-ray and CBC (see Sinusitis). To assess function, consider simple spirometry, pulmonary function studies. To assess therapeutic state, consider theophylline level.

Assess severity, therapeutic needs and asthma education needs. **Differential Diagnosis** bronchiolitis, foreign body aspiration, LTB, bronchitis, pneumonia. **Complications** pulmonary infection, hypoxia, respiratory failure, pneumothorax.

PLAN/MANAGEMENT PROTOCOL
General Measures Explain the nature of asthma to parents and child and give reinforcing literature. Advise allergy proofing (see Allergy Proofing the Bedroom)
　　Ultimately, for the child with persistent symptoms **establish both maintenance and contingency plans.** Carefully construct criteria for use of the latter.

Specific Measures.　　　　　　**ACUTE MEASURES**　　(Consider consultation.)
If pulse less than 140, consider subcut. injection(s) of _____
(BP & P, before and 10 minutes after). Caution patient about expected side effects
　　　　　　　　　　　　　　　or
A nebulizer inhalation of _____ (BP&P as above).
　　　　　　　　　　　and per NIH Guidelines

Consider oral antibiotic Rx _____ *(MIS).

Consider injection of corticosteroid _____ *(MIS).

MAINTENANCE THERAPY
Choose from oral theophylline Rx and/or Rx for inhaled or oral beta adrenergic stimulator _____ *(MIS)
　　　　　　　and per NIH Guidelines (NHLBI's NAEP)
Rx for cromolyn _____ *(MIS)
and/or inhaled corticosteroid _____ *(MIS).
　　　　　　　　　　　and
Consider contingency oral corticosteroid _____ *(MIS).

Note: Do not use sedative tranquilizers, cough suppressants, or antihistamines decongestant combinations without physician consultation. Do consider home Peak Expiratory Flow Rate (PEFR) monitoring.

Physician Consultation. Consider on all newly diagnosed or difficult to manage asthmatics.

Referral. To allergist or pediatric pulmonologist _____.

Immediate Transfer. For severe respiratory distress. Nurse practitioner and physician must define criteria (e.g., pulse above 140) to _____.

Follow-up Plan. After the acute illness in _____ day(s) and when on maint. regime every _____ week(s)/month(s). Monitor serum drug levels as indicated. **Caution parents and child to ask for help if worsening on maintenance therapy and if not helped by contingency plan.**

　　　　　　　　　　　　　　　　　　　　Initials　　Date

*unless allergic, contraindicated,　　　Physician
or pregnant/lactating　　　　　　　　　ARNP

Asthma (Adults)

EVALUATION/DIAGNOSTIC PROTOCOL
<u>Subjective</u>
<u>History</u>. General and respiratory history. Emphasis on history of allergic disorders, both personal and familial. Try to ascertain precipitating factor (infection the most common, but also consider allergy, environmental change, exercise). It is important to assess family history of allergic disorders. Remember that more than 10% of asthmatics may never wheeze but instead have a history of coughing and have been labeled as having recurring acute bronchitis. Obtain meticulous history of medications used in the past 36 hours, including amounts and times taken.

<u>Objective</u>
Physical Examination. General appearance, vital signs, ENT, chest.

Lab. Laboratory tests may not be necessary. For infection, consider chest x-ray and CBC. To assess function, consider simple spirometry or pulmonary function studies. Consider theophylline level.

<u>Assess</u> severity, therapeutic needs and asthma education needs. **Differential Diagnosis.** LTB, bronchitis, pneumonia. **Complications.** Pulmonary infection, hypoxia, respiratory failure, pneumothorax.

PLAN/MANAGEMENT PROTOCOL
General Measures. Explain the nature of asthma to patient and give reinforcing educational literature. Emphasize the need to avoid exposure to all inhalants and tobacco smoke in particular. Advise allergy proofing (<u>see Allergy Proofing</u>). Ultimately, for the adult with persistent symptoms **establish both maintenance and contingency plans.** Carefully construct criteria for use of the latter.

Specific Measures.   **ACUTE MEASURES** (Consider consultation.)
If pulse less than 120, consider subcut. injection(s) of
_____. (Check P and BP, before and 10 minutes after), (caution patient about immediate effects of this injection), or a nebulizer inhalation of _____.
          and per NIH Guidelines
Consider oral antibiotic Rx _____*(MIS).

Consider injection of corticosteroid _____*(MIS).

                MAINTENANCE THERAPY
Choose from oral theophylline Rx and/or Rx for inhaled or oral beta adrenergic stimulator _____*(MIS)
      and per NIH Guidelines (NHLBI's NAEP)
Rx for cromolyn _____*(MIS)
and/or inhaled corticosteroid _____*(MIS).
and/or contingency oral corticosteroid _____*(MIS).

Note: Do not use sedative tranquilizers, cough suppressants, or antihistamines decongestant combinations without physician consultation. Do consider home Peak Expiratory Flow Rate (PEFR) monitoring.

Physician Consultation Consider on all newly diagnosed or difficult to manage asthmatics.

Referral. To allergist or pulmonologist _____.

Immediate Transfer. For severe respiratory distress. Nurse practitioner and physician must define criteria (e.g., pulse above 140 or PEFR) to _____.

Follow-up Plan. After the acute illness in _____ day(s) and when on maint. regime every _____ week(s)/month(s). Monitor serum drug levels as indicated. **Caution patients ask for help if worsening on maintenance therapy.**

                                 Initials   Date

*unless allergic, contraindicated,   Physician
or pregnant/lactating   ARNP

CHAPTER 6
CARDIOVASCULAR

Hypertension, Adults, Initial Visit

EVALUATION/DIAGNOSTIC PROTOCOL

Subjective

History. General medical history and family history. Note that hypertension is usually asymptomatic. Has there been any recent use of medications, prescription or non-prescription, illicit?

Objective

Physical Examination. General appearance, vital signs, retinal, chest, and cardiovascular exam. Be certain your blood pressure reading is not artifactual. If time permits, a more thorough complete physical examination should be performed; otherwise, it should be scheduled. If hypertension confirmed by review of old records, otherwise confirm by serial readings every _____ day(s).

Lab. Consider establishing complete health data base to include chemistry profile, CBC, thyroid profile, lipid profile, EKG, chest x-ray.

Assessment: H. As Defined by Diastolics   Isolated Systolic H.

	Diastolics	Isolated Systolic H.
Borderline	85-89	
Mild	90-104	140-159
Moderate	105-114	160-
Severe	115->	

Differential Diagnosis is directed at etiology with over 90% being idiopathic, better known as "essential" hypertension, which needs to be differentiated from secondary causes. **Complications** include accelerated coronary arterial disease, cardiomyopathy, congestive heart failure, aneurysm, cerebrovascular disease, renal vascular disease.

PLAN/MANAGEMENT PROTOCOL

General Measures. Explain hypertension and its direct relation to shortened life span as well as potential complications if untreated. Provide reinforcing educational materials.

    Begin appropriate habit modification instruction (involve significant family members): weight reduction, sodium restriction, exercise if not contraindicated, discontinuing smoking.

    Outline a program for regular blood pressure monitoring.

Specific Measures. The authors recognize that practice circumstances and patient population may necessitate formulary variation.

Consider an A.C.E. inhibitor _____*(MIS)

                   or

calcium antagonist, _____*(MIS)

                   or

beta blocker _____*(MIS)

                   or

other antihypertensive _____*(MIS).

Physician Consultation. Consider on all newly diagnosed patients, in particular those in the moderate to severely hypertensive range or any with evidence of target organ involvement, consult immediately.

Referral.

Immediate Transfer. Usually not necessary.

Follow-up Plan. Recheck for those on habit modification only every _____ weeks. Recheck blood pressure every _____ day(s) as pharmacotherapy instituted. Otherwise, recheck every _____ week(s) until normotensive.

                                     Initials   Date

* unless allergic, contraindicated,   Physician
or pregnant/lactating   ARNP

Hypertension, Adults, Follow-Up Visit

EVALUATION/DIAGNOSTIC PROTOCOL

Subjective

History. General medical history update. Specific update about how habit modification is progressing. Push the patient for details, reinforcing achievement of goals. Review medication usage and whether or not any side effects have developed.

Objective

Physical Examination. General appearance, vital signs (to include weight, pulse, blood pressure). Consider at some point comparing supine and sitting blood pressures as well as right arm with left arm readings.

Lab. Testing appropriate to drug therapy that has been instituted. Monitor renal function and lipids.

Assessment is directed at determining level of compliance with nondrug programs and compliance with drug therapy. **Complications** are those previously discussed as being the result of hypertension or those known to be associated with the drug therapy employed. Be careful to watch for drug interactions.

PLAN/MANAGEMENT PROTOCOL

General Measures. Again, try to reinforce progress made by the patient habit modification. Also, positively reinforce compliance with pharmacotherapy.

Specific Measures. Change medications if the patient is exhibiting untoward side effects or complications of usage.

Adjust dosage of current medication to bring both systolic and diastolic pressure into the normal range for age. This can be done in a slow, deliberate fashion after several pressure readings have been obtained over weeks or even months, depending upon the nondrug therapy instituted and the patient's success in these areas.

Physician Consultation. Consider on all patients whose pressure remains in the moderate to severely hypertensive range. Similarly, consult immediately for any new evidence or target organ involvement.

Referral.

Immediate Transfer. Usually not necessary.

Follow-up Plan. Recheck blood pressure every _____ week(s) until normotensive. Subsequently recheck every _____ month(s).

	Initials	Date
* unless allergic, contraindicated, or pregnant/lactating	Physician ARNP	

Angina Pectoris

EVALUATION/DIAGNOSTIC PROTOCOL
Subjective
History. Description of the pain, severity, quality, aggravating and alleviating circumstances, duration of each episode, location, radiation, and accompanying symptomatology. Are there predisposing factors: habits (smoking), family history, situational. Are there underlying conditions: diabetes, hypertension, hyper-lipidemia. Note: angina pectoris/myocardial ischemic pain occurs with exertion (or stress) and lasts at least several minutes but not longer than ten. Persistent pain may represent infarct and is an emergency requiring immediate transfer.

Objective
Physical Examination. General appearance, vital signs, chest, musculoskeletal (chest wall) and complete cardiovascular exam. Usually, the angina patient without previous infarct has normal cardiac exam.

Lab. EKG, chest x-ray, chemistry and lipid panels. After consultation additional non-invasive or invasive studies.

Assessment relies on the history. Differential Diagnosis includes myocardial infarction, pulmonary embolus, aortic dissection, and unstable angina which are life-threatening and if being considered then physician consultation and/or immediate transfer is/are indicated. (Also see Acute Chest Pain.) Complications are potentially so serious that physician consultation is necessary.

PLAN/MANAGEMENT PROTOCOL
General Measures. The patient and his/her family must be educated about the nature of coronary artery disease. Emphasize avoiding or altering situations that cause anginal episodes. Habit modification is critical (see Hyperlipidemia and/or Tobacco Abuse). Exercise recommendations should be deferred until diagnostic studies are completed. Underlying conditions must be approached logically. Encourage family and co-workers to learn CPR.

Specific Measures. After Physician Consultation.
                    FOR ACUTE ANGINA
Give Rx nitroglycerin _____*(MIS).
Detailed verbal instructions and cautions to patient and family.
                    PREVENTIVE
Consider Rx long-acting or sustained release nitrate _____*(MIS)
                    and/or
consider Rx beta blocker _____*(MIS)
                    and/or
consider Rx calcium channel blocker _____*(MIS).

Physician Consultation. Consider on all initial presentations, when you have diagnostic uncertainty or follow-up visits with worsening symptoms or signs.

Referral. To cardiologist _____.

Immediate Transfer. As discussed above to _____.

Follow-up Plan. Recheck in _____ week(s) until confident about stability, then less frequently about every _____ months. Caution patient to be seen sooner if worse.

                                              Initials   Date
* unless allergic, contraindicated,   Physician
or pregnant/lactating   ARNP

After Myocardial Infarction

EVALUATION/DIAGNOSTIC PROTOCOL
Subjective
History. Current medical history with attention to any continued chest pain (frequency, severity, quality, aggravating and alleviating circumstances, duration of each episode, location, radiation and accompanying symptomatology) (see also Angina Pectoris), rhythm distrubance, shortness of breath, dyspnea (circumstances). Remember persistent pain or accelerating frequency or progressive intensity may forebode catastrophe.

Objective
Physical Examination. General appearance, vital signs, including weight, chest and lungs, complete cardiovascular (enlarging erratic PMI, gallops, JVD) and abdomen.

Lab. Consider EKG or Gxt, consider chest x-ray. Perform those tests appropriate to current medications. Consider chemistry panel and lipid panel.

Assessment is directed at assessing improved cardiac function or at the least stability. **Differential Diagnosis.** **Complications** include congestive heart failure, recurrent infarcts, aneurysm or chamber rupture, death.

PLAN/MANAGEMENT PROTOCOL
General Measures.
Habit modification is critical (see Hyperlipidemia and/or Tobacco Abuse). Exercise recommendations must be individualized; this can be done by referral to a cardiac rehabilitation program that is supervised. Answer patient and family questions. Bring up for discussion sensitive subjects like resumption of sexual activity. Review the use of all medications. Be sure NTG use is understood and that NTG is fresh.

Specific Measures.   PREVENTIVE
Consider Rx long-acting or sustained release nitrate_____*(MIS)
                                and/or
consider Rx beta blocker _____*(MIS)
                                and/or
consider Rx calcium channel blocker _____*(MIS).

Physician Consultation. For any indication of worsening cardiac function.

Referral.

Immediate Transfer.

Follow-up Plan. Recheck in _____ week(s) until confident about stability and progress. Then recheck every _____ month(s). Caution patient to be seen sooner as needed, setting up specific concerns.

	Initials	Date
* unless allergic, contraindicated,	Physician	
or pregnant/lactating	ARNP	

Congestive Heart Failure

EVALUATION/DIAGNOSTIC PROTOCOL
Subjective
History. General with attention to cardiovascular and pulmonary history (orthopnia, nocturia, proxysmal nocturnal dyspnea). Onset and course of symptoms, aggravating and alleviating factors. Obtain medication and habit history.

Objective
Physical Examination. General appearance, vital signs, including weight, chest (bilateral moist rales), complete cardiovascular (cyanosis, edema, JVD, and S3) and abdominal exam.

Lab. Chest x-ray. Consider EKG, Hgb, electrolyte panel, BUN, creatinine.

Assess severity. **Differential Diagnosis** would include asthma, pulmonary emboli, other pulmonary disease. **Complications**. Arrhythmia, myocardial infarct, or just worsening failure. Be careful of complications from medications.

PLAN/MANAGEMENT PROTOCOL
General Measures. Assess whether or not the patient is already taking the medicines as prescribed. Re-emphasize importance of all medications. Review low sodium diet and hidden sources of dietary sodium. Modest fluid restriction.

Specific Measures.
Induce diuresis with _____*(MIS).

Consider the addition of digoxin _____*(MIS).

Also consider _____*(MIS).
                                          and/or
_____*(MIS).

Physician Consultation. Consider on all new patients, patients not responding to therapy or developing complications.

Referral. Consider consultation with cardiologist.

Immediate Transfer. Should be considered for moderate to severe CHF or obvious acute pulmonary edema.

Follow-up Plan. Follow up in _____ day(s), sooner if worse. Regular follow-up intervals as indicated.

                                                  Initials   Date
* unless allergic, contraindicated,   Physician
or pregnant/lactating   ARNP

Evaluation of Heart Murmurs

The authors find it difficult to construct a detailed narrative protocol confined to a single page and recommend consulting additional references.

EVALUATION/DIAGNOSTIC PROTOCOL
Subjective
History. Previous history of murmur, work-up. Complete medical history, social history, prescription or OTC drug use, exercise history. Specifically, ask about palpitations, chest pain, tachycardia, dizziness, syncope, signs of hyperthyroidism, anemia, or anxiety.

Objective. Complete cardiac exam with attention to careful auscultation noting timing, quality, location, amplitude, radiation and duration. Decide on grade of murmur (Levine and Harvey scale) grade 1, very faint, to grade 6, loudest possible. Also exam carotid, jugular venous, and precordial pulses and heart sounds. Note change in intensity with upright positioning, Valsalva maneuver, presence of clicks or splitting of second sound.

Lab. Unless you are sure this is an innocent murmur, consider CBC, thyroid profile, chemistry panel. Consider EKG and chest x-ray. Consider echocardiography.

Assess whether this is an innocent/physiologic murmur or if the murmur warrants further investigation for underlying cardiac pathology. **Differential Diagnosis**. Systolic-ejection murmurs are frequently noted in otherwise healthy people; they can be grouped into innocent/physiologic murmurs (increased ejection velocity-pregnancy, fever, anemia, hyperthyroidism, exercise or anxiety), and pathologic, including atrial septal defect, aortic regurgitation, bradycardia, aortic stenotic murmurs (aortic stenosis, asymmetric septal hypertrophy, sub- and supravalvular fixed stenosis), pulmonic murmurs (pulmonic stenosis). Pansystolic murmurs are usually pathologic (mitral regurgitation, triscupid regurgitation or ventricular septal defect). Diastolic murmurs also usually indicate pathology (aortic or pulmonic regurgitation or mitral stenosis, atrial or ventricular septal defects). **Complications** are related to presence of underlying cardiac pathology.

PLAN/MANAGEMENT PROTOCOL
General Measures. Explain anatomy and physiology of murmurs to patient or parents. Reassurance if murmur is innocent, explanation of evaluation if indicated. Excessive or unexplained work-up can lead to "cardiac phobia."

Specific Measures. If indicated, for dental and surgical procedure prophylaxsis:

Antibiotic Rx _____ *(MIS)

                                              or

alternative antibiotic Rx _____ *(MIS).

Physician Consultation. As indicated.

Referral. To cardiologist for evaluation when suspecting organic lesion, or
_____ .

Immediate Transfer.

Follow-up Plan. Innocent murmurs, non-cardiac based physiologic murmurs recheck at preventive care exams, or as indicated.

	Initials	Date
* unless allergic, contraindicated, or pregnant/lactating	Physician ARNP	

Mitral Valve Prolapse Syndrome

EVALUATION/DIAGNOSTIC PROTOCOL
Subjective
History. General medical history with attention to cardiovascular and pulmonary history (though most commonly assymptomatic, symptoms may include palpitations irregular or rapid, chest pains, dyspnea, fatigue, or those of a panic attack). Family history. Obtain medication and habits history (tobacco, caffeine, alcohol and other medications prescription or otherwise). Obtain diet and exercise history.

Objective
Physical Examination. General appearance, vital signs, chest, complete cardiovascular (auscultory findings vary from none to mid to late systolic murmer with or without mid to late systolic click(s), and abdomen.

Lab. Consider CBC, chemistry panel, thyroid panel. Consider EKG, chest x-ray. Consider echocardiography.

Assess severity of symptoms and accuracy of diagnosis. **Differential Diagnosis** is directed at differentiating from other valvular disease and other causes of mitral valve disease or underlying pathology creating flow murmers (anemia, thyroid dysfunction, fever) or physiolgic changes (pregnancy, exercise or anxiety). **Complications.**

PLAN/MANAGEMENT PROTOCOL
General Measures. Explain the anatomy of mitral valve prolapse syndrome and usual benignity as regards cardiac physiology. Discuss associated symptomatology. Focus on habits that can be modified to modify symptoms (in particular eliminating nicotine and caffeine). Generally they will feel better eating a well balanced diet, drinking plenty of fluids and getting regular exercise.
    Dental and surgical procedure antibiotic prophylaxis is usually recommended (see specific measures Evaluation of Heart Murmurs).

Specific Measures.
With consultation consider Rx for beta blocker _____*(MIS).

Physician Consultation. All newly diagnosed patients and those with worsening symptoms.

Referral.

Immediate Transfer.

Follow-up Plan. As indicated.

	Initials	Date
* unless allergic, contraindicated,	Physician	
or pregnant/lactating	ARNP	

Evaluation of Arrhythmias

The authors find it difficult to construct a detailed narrative protocol confined to a single page and recommend consulting additional references.

EVALUATION/DIAGNOSTIC PROTOCOL
Subjective
History. Onset and description of symptoms (may be described as pounding, racing, skipping, flopping, or fluttering sensation). Is it isolated beats or continuous when occurring? Associated symptoms. Complete medical history with attention to cardiovascular and pulmonary history. Review use of medications, prescription and otherwise. Review habits (alcohol, caffeine, tobacco). Family history.

Objective
Physical Examination. General appearance, vital signs, orthostatic BP and pulse, skin, thyroid, carotid and jugular venous pulses, chest, cardiovascular exam.

Lab. Usually CBC, chemistry panel, thyroid profile, ECG (may need Holter monitor or telephone monitor). Patient may need to come during an episode. Consider GXT, plasma catecholamine determination (with labile hypertension).

Assess main concern of the patient and level of anxiety. Decide if this is palpitation without arrhythmia. Determine if underlying cardiac disease exists and if arrhythmia is life-threatening. **Differential Diagnosis.** Causes of palpitations without arrhythmias (anxiety, anemia, fever, hyperthyroidism, hypoglycemia, pheochromocytoma, aortic aneurysm, A-V fistula, drugs, aortic regurgitation, aortic stenosis, patent ductus arteriosus, ventral septal defect, cardiomegaly, acute left ventricular failure, tricuspid insufficienty). Superventricular premature beats (atrial and AV junction), atrial premature beats, ventricular premature beats, paroxysmal tachycardias, marked bradycardias, and advanced AV block account for most complaints of palpitation due to arrhythmia. **Complications.** Cardiac neurosis, syncope, shock, death.

PLAN/MANAGEMENT PROTOCOL
General Measures. Respond to patient's concerns when giving reassurance or explaining diagnosis. Ensure patient understands vagal maneuvers properly if recommended. Review use of and side effects of medication. Stress management and relaxation teaching, habit modification, if indicated.

Specific Measures. Usually with consultation. In absence of carotid disease, Valsalva maneuvers and carotid sinus massage may be helpful for supraventricular tachycardia.

Consider _____

_____

Physician Consultation. With diagnostic uncertainty, severe symptoms, or as otherwise indicated.

Referral.

Immediate Transfer. Via ambulance to _____ if condition unstable.

Follow-up Plan. Until diagnosis established, every _____ weeks, then every _____ or as indicated.

	Initials	Date
* unless allergic, contraindicated, or pregnant/lactating	Physician ARNP	

CHAPTER 7
GASTROINTESTINAL

Colic

EVALUATION/DIAGNOSTIC PROTOCOL
Subjective
History. Obtain general history with attention to symptoms (usually abdominal pain and crying), onset (usually starts suddenly), and course (a paroxysm lasting several hours). The pattern is such that it often reoccurs at about the same time of day, usually the evening. Onset of colic is usually in the first month and dissipates in the third month. Are there problems at home? How are the parents coping?

Objective
Physical Examination. Complete physical exam with attention to abdominal exam to differentiate from causes of acute abdomen (see Nontraumatic Abdominal Pain, Children).

Lab. None necessary.

Assess to be certain exam is normal and the history compatible with colic. It is most common for parents to report that an episode ends when the child is either exhausted or has apparent relief with passage of flatus or bowel movement. **Differential Diagnosis** would include causes of acute abdomen, such as malrotation or volvulus in infants under 1 month of age or intussusception. These are emergencies. **Complications.** None.

PLAN/MANAGEMENT PROTOCOL
General Measures. Explain to parents that these episodic periods of fussiness are of unknown cause. Recognize their frustration and remind them that colic is self-limited, usually stopping in the third month. If the patient is one who draws his/her legs up and/or passes gas, then he/she may benefit from simple measures including holding the child upright after eating and burping frequently during the feeding. Sometimes a brief car ride will be helpful as will changing the household routine to give the main caregiver (usually the mother) an opportunity for someone else to take care of the child. In true colic, no diet alteration has proven consistently useful in large studies. Reassure parents, though, there are food intolerances and food allergies that may create similar symptoms. For the nursing child, maternal dietary modification may help; similarly, a formula change may help. Consider referral to parent support group.

Specific Measures. Consider an Rx for _____ *(MIS) or if flatulence is a major symptoms, consider an Rx for _____ *(MIS).

Physician Consultation. For any child who does not have a completely normal exam or exceeds the usual age limits or for parents who do not seem reassured by the process of your evaluation. If suspect potential for abuse.

Immediate Transfer. Only for an acute abdomen.

Follow-up Plan. Remind parents to call again if a fussy episode is prolonged, that is, lasting more than 4 hours, or if a child appears quite ill with vomiting, diarrhea, blood in the bowel movement or fever, which would be signs of something other than a colic paroxysm.

```
                                                    Initials    Date
* unless allergic, contraindicated,      Physician
or pregnant/lactating                    ARNP
```

Gastroenteritis, Infants and Children

EVALUATION/DIAGNOSTIC PROTOCOL

Subjective

History. Sequence of the onset of symptoms, nausea, vomiting, diarrhea, and whether there are signs of bleeding. Description of abdominal pain. Description of bowel movements. Determine whether any OTC or prescription remedies have been used. Briefly review usual dietary habits and, more specifically, any preceding change(s) that might account for this illness. Are there others at home, sitters, or school with similar symptoms? Is this a recurring problem?

Objective

Physical Examination. General appearance, vital signs, ENT, chest, abdominal exam, and when indicated, gloved little finger rectal.

Lab. Stool guaiac during digital exam. Consider also stool for enteric pathogens and ovum and parasites. Recurring illness warrants additional evaluation.

Assess severity and possible etiologies with suspected food contamination or common source outbreak (most commonly viral etiologies, bacterial toxin, bacterial pathogen, protozoan (giardia), and other parasitic infestations). **Differential Diagnosis** would include causes of acute abdomen (see Nontraumatic Abdominal Pain, Infants and Children). **Complications** include volume depletion and electrolyte imbalance. Usually in the recovery phase there are transient food intolerances, such as lactose from lactase deficiency.

PLAN/MANAGEMENT PROTOCOL

General Measures. Remind parents that the best treatment for vomiting is to give their child nothing by mouth for _____ hour(s). This gives the GI tract a rest. Then begin small amounts of clear liquids every 15 minutes for the bottle-fed child. Recommend a specific electrolyte replacement solution _____ or _____. The breast-fed baby can be returned to breast milk when vomiting has not recurred for 12 to 24 hours, then begin re-introducing small amounts of solid foods.

  Diarrhea is treated similar with clear liquids or resumption of nursing, and then advance in a similar fashion. It is prudent to avoid lactose containing products such as milk in these first few days as well as acid fruit juices and spicy foods.

  Review signs of dehydration (sunken eyes, dry skin, decreased urination or dark yellow urine, and more significantly if lethargy or refusal to drink.

  Notify significant appropriate others.

Specific Measures. None for most etiologies.

If giardia, then give Rx _____*(MIS).

Physician Consultation. For all children under _____ months of age. Similarly, consult for children with significant signs of dehydration (approaching or greater than 5% by body weight), those with severe abdominal pain, situations indicative of common source outbreak. Consult immediately for any significant bleeding, or signs or symptoms of shock.

Referral.

Immediate Transfer. If unstable, _____.

Follow-up Plan. Recheck in _____ day(s), if not better, sooner if worse (if the temperature remains over 103°F (39.4°C) or if there is significant blood in the feces or vomitus). Parents should give daily telephone update.

Initials   Date

* unless allergic, contraindicated,   Physician
or pregnant/lactating   ARNP

Gastroenteritis, Adults

EVALUATION/DIAGNOSTIC PROTOCOL

Subjective

History. Sequence onset of symptoms: nausea, vomiting, diarrhea, and whether there are signs of bleeding. Any recent likely causes (family, friends, or co-workers sick, possibly contaminated food, seafood or pond/lake water ingestion)? Description of abdominal pain. Whatever OTC or prescription remedies have been used. Last menstrual period.

Objective

Physical Examination. General appearance, vital signs, abdominal exam, and rectal.

Lab. Stool guaiac during digital exam. Consider also stool for enteric pathogens and ova and parasites.

Assess severity and possible etiologies with suspected food contamination or common source outbreak (most commonly viral etiologies, bacterial toxin, bacterial pathogen, protozoan (giardia), and other parasitic infestations). **Differential Diagnosis** would include irritable bowel syndrome and the inflammatory bowel disorders. **Complications.** Volume depletion, electrolyte imbalance, and shock.

PLAN/MANAGEMENT PROTOCOL

General Measures.

Nothing by mouth for _____ hours.
Then begin clear liquid diet for _____ hours.
Then advance to _____.
Notify significant appropriate others.

Specific Measures.

Consider anti-diarrheal OTC/Rx _____*(MIS)

and/or

consider anti-nauseant Rx _____*(MIS).

If giardia, then give Rx _____*(MIS).

Physician Consultation. Consider for severity evidenced by signs of dehydration (5% or greater by weight), such as tachycardia, postural hypotension or for significant bleeding or for marked abdominal pain or marked tenderness or for recurrent or persistent symptomatology.

Referral.

Immediate Transfer. If unstable, _____.

Follow-up Plan. In _____ days(s) (could be telephonic), if no better, sooner if worse.

	Initials	Date
Physician		
ARNP		

* unless allergic, contraindicated, or pregnant/lactating

Constipation, Infants and Children

EVALUATION/DIAGNOSTIC PROTOCOL

Subjective

History. General and GI history with specific attention to stool characteristics, size, consistency, and frequency. Any bleeding? Obtain dietary history and recent use of medications, prescription or otherwise.

Objective

Physical Examination. General appearance, vital signs, ENT, chest, cardiovascular, abdomen, with gloved little finger rectal exam optional.

Lab. Stool guaiac with rectal exam. For infants, be certain to review their neonatal thyroid function test.

Assess severity and distinguish between acute and chronic onset. **Differential Diagnosis.** Dietary change, recent acute illness, change in toilet routine, emotional stress, drug side effects, metabolic (cystic fibrosis) and endocrine causes, neurogenic, and anatomic. **Complications** include fecal impaction/incontinence/obstruction, anal fissure, behavioral and emotional problems (affecting the family, too).

PLAN/MANAGEMENT PROTOCOL

General Measures. Reassure parents that it's usually easy to treat an infant's or child's constipation. Increase the amount of fluid in the infant or child's diet. Babies who have begun solids may be switched to barley cereal or given a teaspoon or two of pureed prunes each day. Older children may be given age appropriate equivalents, in particular plenty of fruits, vegetables, and especially bran and bran products. Emphasize to the older child the need to increase the amount of fluids he/she drinks. Remind the older child to respond to the "urge to go" by heading for the toilet. Consider using behavior modification techniques such as "star charts" to encourage regular bowel habits.

Specific Measures.

In infants, consider _____ *(MIS).

In older children, as a fiber supplement, consider _____ *(MIS)
or consider _____ *(MIS).

Physician Consultation. Consider for any infant or child in considerable distress or where there is a likely fecal impaction. Similarly, consider for cases of chronic constipation.

Referral.

Immediate Transfer. Consider for impaction or obstruction to _____.

Follow-up Plan. In _____ days, sooner if worse.

	Initials	Date
* unless allergic, contraindicated,	Physician	
or pregnant/lactating	ARNP	

Constipation in Adults

EVALUATION/DIAGNOSTIC PROTOCOL
Subjective
History. General history and GI history specific attention to stool characteristics, size, consistency, and stool frequency (if alternating, see <u>Irritable Bowel Syndrome</u>). Any bleeding? Weight change? Obtain dietary history. Recent usage of OTC medications and complete medication history. Family history.

Objective
Physical Examination. General appearance, vital signs, abdominal exam, rectal exam.

Lab. Stool guaiac with rectal exam. Consider CBC, chemistry screening battery, and thyroid function tests (including TSH). Recommend flexible sigmoidoscopy, if appropriate.

Assess whether acute or chronic and potential for underlying pathology. **Differential diagnosis.** Look for dietary change, drug use or abuse (prescription or non-prescription, including laxatives, narcotic analgesics, anticolinergics, certain antiacids), metabolic or endocrine causes, neurogenic, neoplastic and anatomic. **Complications** include fecal impaction, hemorrhoids or rectal fissures.

PLAN/MANAGEMENT PROTOCOL
General Measures. Review specific dietary changes, in particular increasing high fiber foods (or supplements), increasing water intake. Daily exercise, too, is helpful. Recommend daily regular elimination time.

Specific Measures.
Specific recommendation of fiber supplement _____ *(MIS)
or
consider OTC or Rx stool softener _____ *(MIS)
and possibly
consider stimulant/laxative _____ *(MIS).

Physician Consultation. Consider for positive stool guaiac, severe abdominal pain and/or suspected acute abdomen. Later consultation if underlying condition requires additional treatment or further delineation. Also for failure to respond to therapy. In patients over 50, if symptoms have recently developed.

Referral.

Immediate Transfer. Usually not necessary unless acute abdomen suspected.

Follow-up Plan. In _____ days/weeks/months, sooner if worse.

Initials   Date
* unless allergic, contraindicated,   Physician
or pregnant/lactating   ARNP

Irritable Bowel Syndrome

EVALUATION/DIAGNOSTIC PROTOCOL
<u>Subjective</u>
History. General, dietary, and gastrointestinal history, onset and course of symptoms. Ascertain use of medications, amount of caffeine consumption, smoking history, alcohol use and level of stress. Classically, these patients have frequent loose stools with no bleeding and often mucus.

<u>Objective</u>
Physical Examination. General appearance, vital signs (include weight), abdominal, and rectal exam.

Lab. Stool guaiac. Consider additional GI tests, including stool for O&P, stool for enteric pathogen, radiographic studies and/or endoscopy. Consider CBC, Chemistry Panel and amylase.

<u>**Assess**</u> severity of patient's symptoms. **Differential Diagnosis** includes peptic ulcer disease, the inflammatory and infectious gastroenteridities, food intolerances (lactose) and allergies, diverticulitis (see <u>Diverticulitis</u>), pancreatic disorders and intraabdominal neoplasm. IBS is a diagnosis of exclusion. **Complications** considerable psychologic and social ramifications but by definition no serious physiologic sequelae.

<u>**PLAN/MANAGEMENT PROTOCOL**</u>
General Measures. Explain the nature of irritable bowel syndrome, and that it is a diagnosis of exclusion, that modifying the symptoms usually requires habit modification. Remind patients to eat regular meals, taking enough time to eat and chew slowly.

High bulk diets are very helpful. If the patient is not amenable to dietary bulk, consider a fiber supplement _____. With the supplement, patient needs to be reminded that plenty of liquids are important to the diet.

The patient may want to avoid stimulant liquids, such as all caffeinated beverages, carbonated beverages, and too much fruit juice. Caution patients to avoid foods that do seem to consistently cause symptoms. Discuss stress, coping behaviors such as regular exercise and relaxation techniques.

Specific Measures. Consider prescribing an antispasmodic _____*(MIS).

Physician Consultation. Consider for newly diagnosed, severe symptomatology or lack of therapeutic response. Specifically, consult about unexpected positive test results.

Referral.

Immediate Transfer. Usually not necessary.

Follow-up Plan. Recheck patient in _____ week(s), sooner if worse.

	Initials	Date
* unless allergic, contraindicated,	Physician	
or pregnant/lactating	ARNP	

Diverticulosis & Diverticulitis

EVALUATION/DIAGNOSTIC PROTOCOL
Subjective
History. Detailed description of pain beginning with characteristics and location at onset and subsequently, aggravating and alleviating factors, radiating and accompanying symptomatology (general, gastrointestinal, genitourinary). Previous similar symptomatology. General medical and surgical history. Review habits, in particular dietary practices, caffeine and alcohol intake. Any use of drugs over the counter or prescription.

Objective
Physical Examination. General appearance, vital signs, oropharyngeal, chest, cardiovascular, abdomen (pelvic), rectal.

Lab. Stool guaiac. Consider CBC, _____. Consider when not acute radiographic studies _____ and/or consider endoscopy.

Assessment is directed at severity and potential underlying pathology, the **Differential Diagnosis.** Includes infectious and inflammatory gastroenteridities, irritable bowel syndrome, mechanical obstruction (from stictures to entrapments to infarcts) (see also Constipation, Adults), and most significantly neoplasms. **Complications.** Obstruction, perforation, hemorrhage.

PLAN/MANAGEMENT PROTOCOL
General Measures. Explain the condition (use illustrations) and its relation to highly refined diets. (During ACUTE diverticulitis only a clear liquid diet is appropriate). Review food groups high in fiber giving specific suggestions acceptable to the patient also review those foods to be avoided because of potential to inflame diverticuli (nuts, corn, popcorn, seedy fruit [strawberries, raspberries, figs, grapes], other tiny seed [poppy, carraway]). Promote healthful eating habits, meals at regular intervals, eating and chewing slowly, drinking plenty of liquids. Promote healthful bowel habits and the value of regular exercise. Distribute educational materials.

Specific Measures   **ACUTE MEASURES** (Consider physician consultation.)
If hospitalization not required institute oral antibiotic Rx _____*(MIS).

NON-ACUTE MEASURES
Long term consider adding a fiber supplement _____*(MIS).
and consider adding stool softener _____*(MIS)

Physician Consultation. For positive stool guiac, severe abdominal pain and/or suspected acute abdomen. Also for diagnostic uncertainty. Later consultation for failure to respond to therapy.

Referral.

Immediate Transfer. For acute abdomen.

Follow-up Plan. Initially in _____ days/weeks and then every _____ months or as needed.

Initials   Date

* unless allergic, contraindicated,   Physician
or pregnant/lactating   ARNP

Hiatal Hernia &
Reflux Esophagitis

EVALUATION/DIAGNOSTIC PROTOCOL
Subjective
History. Onset, course, description of pain (have patient define "indigestion" and "heartburn"), aggravating or alleviating factors, location, radiating symptomatology. Previous history of similar symptoms, evaluations and treatments. General medical history. Review use of medications, prescription and otherwise. Review habits, in particular dietary practices, smoking history, alcohol intake. Any current stressors?

Objective
Physical Examination. General appearance, vital signs, oropharyngeal, chest, cardiac, abdominal and rectal exam.

Lab. Stool guaiac, CBC, other lab _____. Consider radiographic studies (barium swallow/upper GI) and/or intraesophageal pH or more commonly endoscopy referral. Also consider ultrasound and oral cholecystogram.

Assessment is directed at documenting reflux, its severity and chronicity as well as etiology (true hiatal hernia, esophageal motility disorders). **Differential Diagnosis** includes peptic ulcer disease, pancreatitis, cholecystic disease, myocardial infarct, aortic dissection and neoplasms. **Complications**. Strictures, ulceration (hemorrhage and perforation).

PLAN/MANAGEMENT PROTOCOL
General Measures. Explain the anatomy and physiology of reflux and/or hiatal hernia. Promote healthful habits decrease or stop tobacco use, caffeine, and alcohol, and reduce weight if needed. Stop any food they know are bothersome and stop medications that aggravate the problem (aspirin, ibuprofen, etc.). Institute measures to reduce reflux pressure including, eating more frequent smaller meals during the day, avoiding eating at least several hours prior to bed, avoid bending and stooping after eating, avoid clothes which are tight on the abdomen, and consider having the patient elevate the head of their bed.

Specific Measures
Recommend use of an antacid_____*(MIS)
                                  and/or
consider an Rx for an H2 antagonist_____*(MIS)
                                  and/or
consider an Rx for a GI motility stimulant _____*(MIS).

Physician Consultation. Consider for severe symptomotology or lack of therapeutic response. Consider also before discontinuing prescribed aggravating medications.

Referral.

Immediate Transfer. Usually not necessary unless suspecting an emergent etiology.

Follow-up Plan. Initially in _____ week(s) and then every _____ month(s) or as needed.

	Initials	Date
* unless allergic, contraindicated, or pregnant/lactating	Physician ARNP	

Peptic Ulcer Disease

EVALUATION/DIAGNOSTIC PROTOCOL
Subjective
History. Onset, course, description of pain, aggravating or alleviating factors, radiating symptomatology. Previous history of similar symptoms, definite peptic ulcer disease, definite hiatal hernia. Review use of medications, prescription and otherwise. Review habits, in particular dietary practices, smoking history, alcohol intake.

Objective
Physical Examination. General appearance, vital signs, abdominal and rectal exam.

Lab. Stool guaiac, CBC, Chemistry Panel, serum amylase. Consider radiographic studies (upper GI series, cholecystogram or ultrasound) or endoscopy referral.

Assessment. Severity may provide a clue to underlying pathology. **Differential Diagnosis** would include reflux esophagitis (see Hiatal Hernia), pancreatitis, cholecystic disease, hepatic diseases, aortic dissection, myocardial infarct, and neoplasms. **Complications.** Obstruction, perforation, hemorrhage.

PLAN/MANAGEMENT PROTOCOL
General Measures. Explain to the patient the nature of indigestion and the potential complications if left untreated.

Treatment involves eating regular meals, eliminating use of gastrointestinal irritants, particularly aspirin and other anti-inflammatories. Similarly, caffeine should be limited or eliminated. Caution the smoker about this habit's contribution to increased risk of complications.

Remind patient that this can be a recurrent problem and require retreatment.

Specific Measures.
Recommend use of an antacid _____*(MIS)
                                                    or
give an Rx for H2 histamine antagonist _____*(MIS)
                                                    or

alternative Rx _____*(MIS)
                                                    or
alternative Rx _____*(MIS).

Physician Consultation. Consider for severely ill, active bleeding, or for diagnostic uncertainty.

Referral.

Immediate Transfer. For severe bleed or acute abdomen to
_____.

Follow-up Plan. Office visit every _____ week(s) until improving, then every _____ week(s) for _____ week(s), sooner if worse. After diagnosis established and symptoms improved then follow-up every _____ weeks.

	Initials	Date
* unless allergic, contraindicated, or pregnant/lactating	Physician ARNP	

Hemorrhoids

EVALUATION/DIAGNOSTIC PROTOCOL
<u>Subjective</u>
History. Determine whether acute or chronic. Obtain patient's description of bleeding, pain, aggravating and alleviating circumstances. Review bowel habits and general physical habits as these are likely contributing factors in developing of these varices.

<u>Objective</u>
Physical Examination. General appearance, vital signs, rectal exam (inspection, palpation, and then digital exam). Consider anoscopy.

Lab. Usually none necessary.

<u>Assess</u> severity, need for surgical intervention. **Differential Diagnosis.** Need to distinguish acute thrombosis from protruding internal hemorrhoids, abscess, fistula, condyloma. **Complications** are bleeding, pain, abscess.

PLAN/MANAGEMENT PROTOCOL
General Measures. Explain the nature of hemorrhoids, in particular emphasizing to the patient that these are vascular lesions, the result of practices, habits, or constipation, which increase anal rectal pressure.

If in acute pain, limit activity. Prone position provides most relief. Encourage frequent sitz baths for 20-30 minutes at least 3 times a day.

Discuss improved diet fiber content and increased fluid intake. Discuss anal hygiene after defecation.

Specific Measures.
Consider bulking agent _____ *(MIS)
and/or
consider stool softener _____ *(MIS)
and/or
consider treatment with cream, suppository, or foam, Rx _____ *(MIS).

Physician Consultation. Consider for acutely thrombosed hemorrhoids being seen within the first 24 hours or for severe bleeding. Also consider for persistent or worsening symptomatology if therapy outlined above has been tried.

Referral.

Immediate Transfer.

Follow-up Plan. Recheck in _____ days if not improved, sooner if worse.

	Initials	Date
* unless allergic, contraindicated,	Physician	
or pregnant/lactating	ARNP	

Anal Fissures

EVALUATION/DIAGNOSTIC PROTOCOL

Subjective

History. Determine whether the complaint is acute or chronic. Obtain patient's description of the pain, aggravating or alleviating circumstances, and whether or not it is accompanied by bleeding or purulent discharge. Review bowel habits, sexual habits, and general exercise and eating habits. This is the most common cause of rectal bleeding.

Objective

Physical Examination. General appearance, vital signs, rectal exam (inspection, palpation, and then gloved digital exam). Consider anoscopy.

Lab. Usually none necessary.

Assess as to whether this is an acute or chronic problem, its severity, and the implication for favorable response to conservative treatment. **Differential Diagnosis** is directed at assuring yourself of the diagnosis as fissure rather than fistula or abscess. Chronic fissures or fistulas may be associated with inflammatory bowel disorders. **Complications** are perirectal abscess. More common is a change in bowel habits because of painful defecation.

PLAN/MANAGEMENT PROTOCOL

General Measures. Explain the nature of anal fissure to the patient, in particular emphasizing that it is a tear in the lining of the anal canal. If the patient is in acute pain, limit activity, encourage frequent sitz baths for 20-30 minutes 3 times a day. Discuss improved fiber diet content, increase fluid intake. Discuss anal hygiene after defecation. Address issue of risk for AIDS as appropriate.

Specific Measures.

Consider bulking agent _____ *(MIS)

and/or

consider stool softener _____ *(MIS)

and/or

consider treatment with cream, suppository, or foam, Rx _____ *(MIS).

Physician Consultation. Consider for severe pain or bleeding or suspected underlying or predisposing condition. Similarly, consult for any that has not improved with therapy.

Referral.

Follow-up Plan. Recheck in _____ days if not improved, sooner if worse.

	Initials	Date
Physician		
ARNP		

* unless allergic, contraindicated, or pregnant/lactating

CHAPTER 8
RENAL UROLOGIC

Urinary Tract Infection, Children

EVALUATION/DIAGNOSTIC PROTOCOL

Subjective

History. General and urologic history. Recognize that in children UTI can be asymptomatic. Or in addition to or instead of typical urinary tract symptomatology, symptoms may be vague or non-localized, including general symptoms (fever, irritability, lethargy, nausea, anorexia) or more localized (such as any abdominal pain). Family history (polycystic disease).

Objective

Physical Examination. General appearance, vital signs, ENT, neck, chest, cardio-vascular, abdominal (CVA tenderness, suprapubic tenderness), and genital exam.

Lab. Urinalysis (pyuria is not diagnostic) and urine culture (consider sensitivities). Appropriate attention should be given to the method of collection to obtain clean-catch, midstream, or straight cath specimen. Consider renal and pelvic ultrasonography immediately in a severely ill child and/or radiographic studies, voiding cystourethrography and intravenous pyelography 3-6 weeks after resolution of the infection in all males and in females under 5 years of age after the initial infection. Similar studies should be performed in females with recurrent infection.

Assessment is directed at establishing definite bacteriuria. The standard is 100,000 organisms per milliliter. Even a count of 10,000 to 100,000 may indicate significant bacteriuria. **Differential Diagnosis.** Genital tract infections and pinworms. **Complications** are septicemia, renal damage.

PLAN/MANAGEMENT PROTOCOL

General Measures. Review urinary tract anatomy with the family and/or the patient. If the patient is female, remind them that this structural difference results in an incidence of infection over 10 times that in males. Discuss habit and hygiene modification. Encourage daily bathing but using non-irritating soap. Bubble baths should be discontinued. Parents should wipe the infant female from front to back. The older child can do it herself. Emphasize the high incidence of recurrence amongst females. Discuss the concept of asymptomatic infection and the need for close follow-up.

Encourage plenty of fluids and frequent urination.

Specific Measures.

Treat with antibiotic Rx _____ *(MIS)

or

alternative antibiotic, consider _____ *(MIS).

Physician Consultation. On all infants under _____ months and on all males. Immediate consultation is necessary in the toxic appearing, severely pained, or vomiting child.

Referral.

Immediate Transfer.

Follow-up Plan. The child should be re-examined in _____ days, sooner if worse, or if persistent vomiting or unable to hold down fluids. Arrangements should be made for a follow-up urinalysis during the infection in _____ days and/or after the infection is resolved, _____ days later with a repeat urine culture. Serial urine cultures should be arranged subsequently every _____ weeks or every _____ months.

	Initials	Date
* unless allergic, contraindicated, or pregnant/lactating	Physician ARNP	

Cystitis, Men

EVALUATION/DIAGNOSTIC PROTOCOL

Subjective

History. General, sexual, and genitourinary history. Review of symptoms, course, potentiating factors and precipitating events.

Objective

Physical Examination. General appearance, vital signs, abdominal, genital, and prostate exam.

Lab. Urinalysis and culture. Consider sensitivities of a midstream clean-catch specimen. Consider prostatic secretion analysis and chlamydia culture.

Assess severity and its implication for favorable response to therapy. **Differential Diagnosis** includes other sites of infection in the male urinary tract and serious consideration must be given to underlying pathology as true cystitis is uncommon in males (see Pyelonephritis, Adults, Acute Prostatitis, Epididymitis and sections covering Male STDs). **Complications** not likely unless there is significant underlying pathology.

PLAN/MANAGEMENT PROTOCOL

General Measures. Encourage patients to force fluids and to consider urinating a bit more frequently, making every effort to completely empty the bladder. Encourage voiding shortly after intercourse. When appropriate, recommend partner(s) be evaluated for infection.

Specific Measures.
Treat with a 10-14 day course of _____ *(MIS)
                                              or
consider as an alternative _____ *(MIS).

Some will benefit from urinary tract analgesic dye Rx _____ *(MIS).

Physician Consultation. Consider for septicemia or toxicity, severe pain, or significant retention. Similarly, consider consulting for patients with potentiating factors or underlying conditions.

Referral.

Immediate Transfer.

Follow-up Plan. In _____ days, sooner if worse. If improving, consider follow-up urine culture _____ days after antibiotic therapy completed.

	Initials	Date
* unless allergic, contraindicated,	Physician	
or pregnant/lactating	ARNP	

Pyelonephritis, Men

EVALUATION/DIAGNOSTIC PROTOCOL
Subjective
History. General medical and urinary with review of symptoms, course, potentiating factors and precipitating events. Previous urologic procedures. Recent medications.

Objective
Physical Examination. General appearance, vital signs, abdominal, genital, and prostate exam.

Lab. Urinalysis with culture and sensitivities. Consider ultrasonic or radiographic studies.

Assess severity and its implication for favorable response to therapy. **Differential Diagnosis** includes other sites of infection in the male urinary tract and serious consideration must be given to underlying pathology as true pyelonephritis is uncommon in males (see Nephrolithiasis, Adults, sections covering Male STDs). **Complications** in part depend on presence of significant underlying pathology, but include; chronic infection, renal damage, sepsis.

PLAN/MANAGEMENT PROTOCOL
General Measures. Encourage patients to force fluids and to expect to urinate more frequently. Emphasize the relative infrequency of this problem in men and the necessity for further evaluation and follow-up.

Specific Measures. Treat with an oral antibiotic for 10-14 days.
Initial Rx _____*(MIS)
or
consider as an alternative _____*(MIS).

Physician Consultation. Consider for severe infection, septicemia or toxicity, severe pain, Similarly, consider consulting for patients with potentiating factors or underlying conditions.

Referral.

Immediate Transfer. Per physician to _____.

Follow-up Plan. In _____ days, sooner if worse. Consider follow-up urine culture _____ days after antibiotic therapy completed.

	Initials	Date
* unless allergic, contraindicated, or pregnant/lactating	Physician ARNP	

Nephrolithiasis

EVALUATION/DIAGNOSTIC PROTOCOL
<u>Subjective</u>
History. Description of the pain or change in location, aggravating or alleviating factors, radiation and accompanying symptomatology. Past history of calculi or family history. Obtain dietary and drug history. (Classically severe unilateral pain/"colic," so severe that the patient is agitated and diaphoretic.)

<u>Objective</u>
Physical Examination. General appearance, vital signs, abdomen, genitalia and back.

Lab. Urinalysis and culture (classically shows RBCs in marked disproportion to WBCs). Urine should be examined for crystals and sediment. Serum calcium and uric acid. Consider emergency IVP in patients in particular without compatible past medical history. Definitely send stone for analysis when available.

<u>Assess</u> severity and its implication for favorable outpatient management. Differential **Diagnosis** includes pyelonephritis, epididymitis, testicular torsion, strangulated hernia, acute salpingitis, ectopic pregnancy, ovarian cyst, appendicitis, diverticulitis, intestinal obstruction, intestinal infarction, peptic ulcer disease, pancreatitis, cholecystic disease, herpes zoster, musculoskeletal pain. Complications. Secondary infection and renal damage.

PLAN/MANAGEMENT PROTOCOL
General Measures. In those in whom outpatient management seems favorable, encourage increased fluid intake on the order of 8-16 glasses per 24 hours. Recommend rest. Meticulously instruct the patient in the process of filtering the urine to collect the stone should it pass. Drip coffee filters are ideal for this purpose, or pharmacies have special filters for sale.

Specific Measures. If diagnostically confident and/or with physician's approval, administer analgesic injection _____, usually in combination with _____.

Prescribe oral narcotic analgesic _____ *(MIS).
Consider oral antibiotic _____ *(MIS).

Long-term, consider prophylactic Rx _____ *(MIS).

Physician Consultation. Consider for patients in severe pain. Mandatory consultation for those whose diagnosis remains unclear or who are toxic appearing or medically unstable. Consider also if not improved in 12-24 hours.

Referral.

Immediate Referral. For toxic-appearing, medically unstable, or intractable pain.

Follow-up Plan. In _____ hours, sooner if worsening pain or vomiting interfering with oral hydration. Long-term at regular intervals.

	Initials	Date
* unless allergic, contraindicated, or pregnant/lactating	Physician ARNP	

Acute Prostatitis

EVALUATION/DIAGNOSTIC PROTOCOL
Subjective
History. General, genitourinary, and sexual history. Onset and course of pain (may be referred to abdomen, lower back, or thighs), aggravating and alleviating factors. Recent use of OTC and prescription medications.

Objective
Physical Examination. General appearance, vital signs, abdomen, genitalia, including prostate.

Lab. Urinalysis, prostatic secretion microscopic. Consider culture and sensitivity. Consider chlamydia culture.

Assess severity. **Differential Diagnosis** includes UTI, epididymitis, prostatic carcinoma, prostatodynia, rectal abscess, low back pain. **Complications** are acute urinary retention, chronic prostatitis.

PLAN/MANAGEMENT PROTOCOL
General Measures. Bed rest, lots of fluid, hot tub baths 30 minutes three times a day. OTC analgesic or anti-inflammatory. Discontinue all OTC (consider discontinuing Rx's) with anticolinergic properties such as antihistamine decongestants.

Specific Measures.
Rx for oral antibiotic _____*(MIS)
                                              or
alternative oral antibiotic _____*(MIS).

Physician Consultation. Consider for high fever, retention, other evidence of bacteremia. Also for underlying or predisposing conditions.

Referral. Consider for frequent recurrences, to urologist _____.

Immediate Transfer. For acute retention.

Follow-up Plan. Recheck in _____ days or sooner if no better or if worsening.

Initials   Date
* unless allergic, contraindicated,   Physician
or pregnant/lactating   ARNP

Epididymitis

EVALUATION/DIAGNOSTIC PROTOCOL

Subjective

History. General, genitourinary, sexual history. If the patient has scrotal pain, obtain description of onset and course, if there is radiation and what are the aggravating or alleviating factors, previous history of urinary or genital tract infection.

Objective

Physical Examination. General, vital signs, abdomen, genital, prostate.

Lab. Urinalysis and culture. Consider sensitivities. If urethral discharge, then smear, chlamydial and GC culture.

Assessment of severity and likely etiology. Be aware that there is often history of changed or increased physical activity. **Differential Diagnosis** from testicular torsion, varicoele, spermatocoele, scrotal abscess, testicular tumor. It should be simple to distinguish from a hernia, but could be difficult to distinguish from a hydrocele. **Complications** include chronic epididymitis. Again, any mass persisting at follow-up should be evaluated by a urologist.

PLAN/MANAGEMENT PROTOCOL

General Measures. Explain the anatomy of the genitourinary tract, the degree of limitation of activity directly related to the degree of discomfort. Increased scrotal support is helpful.

Specific Measures.
Consider antibiotic Rx _____*(MIS)
or
alternative antibiotic consider _____*(MIS).

Usually prescribe an N.S.A.I.D. _____*(MIS).

Physician Consultation. Consider for a patient with severe discomfort, intolerant of oral medications, potentially unstable, or emotionally in need of an additional opinion.

Referral.

Immediate Transfer. With suspicion of testicular torsion.

Follow-up Plan. In _____ days, sooner, if worse.

		Initials	Date
* unless allergic, contraindicated,	Physician		
or pregnant/lactating	ARNP		

Benign Prostatic Hypertrophy

EVALUATION/DIAGNOSTIC PROTOCOL
Subjective
History. General, genitourinary, and sexual history. Onset and course of symptoms, aggravating and alleviating factors. Current medications.

Objective
Physical Examination. General appearance, vital signs, abdomen, genital including prostate.

Lab. Urinalysis with microscopic, urine C and S. Consider serum chemistry to include BUN and creatinine. Consider acid phosphatase and prostatic specific antigen (PSA).

Assess severity of symptoms and of obstruction. **Differential Diagnosis**. Acute prostatitis (bacterial, inflammatory, prostatodynia), prostatic carcinoma. **Complications** are acute urinary retention, obstruction, and secondary infection.

PLAN/MANAGEMENT PROTOCOL
General Measures. Explain to the patient the nature of the prostate, and when nonbacterial in origin that this often is a condition that requires surgery. Provide or recommend educational materials (such as The Prostate Book from Consumer Reports).
Consider discontinuing all medications with anticholenergic properties.

Specific Measures.
If suspect chronic bacterial cause, give Rx _____*(MIS)

or refer to consulting urologist _____.

Physician Consultation. For diagnostic uncertainty.

Immediate Referral. For acute retention/obstruction.

Follow-up Plan. Every _____ months, sooner if worse, or per urologic consultant.

Initials   Date

* unless allergic, contraindicated,
or pregnant/lactating

Physician
ARNP

Non-specific Urethritis

EVALUATION/DIAGNOSTIC PROTOCOL

Subjective

History. Description of symptoms, sequencing with onset of discharge. Genitourinary and sexual history (known chlamydial contact).

Objective

Physical Examination. Vital signs, general appearance, genital and rectal exam.

Lab. Wet prep or gram stain of discharge and urethral (chlamydia) culture (in some instances rectal discharge culture). Gonorrhea culture, and consider RPR/VDRL, HIV.

Assessment is directed at determining the presence of other STDs and insuring treatment of all contacts. **Differential Diagnosis** includes the other STDs. Recognize that many patients have more than one STD. **Complications** include prostatitis and epididymitis, as well as social ramifications.

PLAN/MANAGEMENT PROTOCOL

General Measures. Explain the confusing terminology that surrounds this illness, and in fact that the causative organism is known and that finding it does not preclude the presence of other STDs for which additional investigation is usually warranted. Advise abstinence until the patient and partner(s) are fully treated and follow-up culture is negative. Report to Public Health Department. Strongly recommend routine use of condoms.

Specific Measures.
Treat with a tetracycline antibiotic _____ *(MIS)

or

alternative Rx, use erythromycin Rx _____ *(MIS).

Physician Consultation. Consider if the diagnosis remains unclear or patient is emotionally unstable. Similarly, consider consultation at follow-up if the patient has refractory symptomatology.

Referral.

Follow-up Plan. Repeat chlamydia culture in _____ days/weeks. Recheck sooner if worse. Re-emphasize the need for abstinence.

	Initials	Date
* unless allergic, contraindicated, or pregnant/lactating	Physician ARNP	

Gonococcal Urethritis

EVALUATION/DIAGNOSTIC PROTOCOL
<u>Subjective</u>
History. Description of symptoms, sequencing with onset of discharge. Genito-urinary and sexual history (known contact). Note: Incubation period is 3-14 days and that 10% of males and 75% of females are asymptomatic.

<u>Objective</u>
Physical Examination. Vital signs, general appearance, oral, genital and rectal exam.

Lab. Wet prep or gram stain of discharge and/or urethral discharge culture (in some instances rectal discharge or oropharyngeal culture). Chlamydial culture. Consider VDRL/RPR, HIV.

<u>Assessment</u> is directed at determining the presence of other STDs and insuring treatment of all contacts. **Differential Diagnosis** includes the other STDs. Recognize that many patients have more than one STD. **Complications** are unlikely, except as relates to social ramifications.

PLAN/MANAGEMENT PROTOCOL
General Measures. Explain this illness,and that finding it does not preclude the presence of other STDs for which additional investigation is usually warranted. Advise abstinence until the patient and partners are fully treated and follow-up culture is negative. Report to Public Health Department. Suggest employing condoms in the future.

Specific Measures. Treat according to the most recent C.D.C. recommendations. Currently, <u>Ceftriaxone 250mg I.M. once</u> (MIS) is that drug of choice.

If contraindicated, or as alternate Rx _____*(MIS)

or

consider additional Rx for N.G.U. too _____*(MIS).

Physician Consultation. Consider if the diagnosis remains unclear or patient is emotionally unstable. Similarly, consider consultation at follow-up if the patient has refractory symptomatology.

Referral.

Immediate Transfer Usually not necessary.

Follow-up Plan. Repeat gonorrhea culture in _____ days. Recheck sooner if worse. Re-emphasize the need for abstention.

	Initials	Date
* unless allergic, contraindicated,	Physician	
or pregnant/lactating	ARNP	

Syphilis, Males

EVALUATION/DIAGNOSTIC PROTOCOL

Subjective

History. Description of symptoms, sequencing with development of sore. Genitourinary and sexual history (known exposure to syphilis). Note: Primary stage--incubation period is 9-90 days; secondary stage is 3-8 weeks after chancre is healed (this usually occurs after 2-6 weeks).

Objective

Physical Examination. Vital signs, general appearance, genital and rectal exam.

Lab. Dark field examination if available. VDRL/RPR. Confirm with FTA-ABS. Consider testing for co-existing STDs, including HIV.

Assessment is directed at determining the presence of other STDs and insuring treatment of all contacts (who are they?). **Differential Diagnosis** includes the other STDs and other causes of skin ulcers including herpes and chancroid. Secondary lues macular papular dermatitis that is intermittently symptomatic and has a large differential diagnosis (mononucleosis, pityriasis rosea, and the coxsackie viruses). Again, recognize that many patients have more than one STD. **Complications** include cardiovascular disease, central nervous system damage including blindness, bone disease.

PLAN/MANAGEMENT PROTOCOL

General Measures. Patient education concerning this disease, course and outcome. Emphasize the importance of notifying sexual contacts. Advise abstinence until the patient and partners are fully treated and follow-up culture is negative. Report to Public Health Department. Strongly recommend routine use of condoms.

Specific Measures. Treat according to the most recent CDC recommendations.

PRIMARY, SECONDARY, or LATENT of LESS THAN 1 YEAR
Currently, <u>Benzathine Penicillin G 2.4 million units I.M.</u> *(MIS).
Consider alternative Rx _____ *(MIS)
or
consider alternative Rx _____ *(MIS).

LATENT of MORE THAN 1 YEAR
Currently, <u>Benzathine Penicillin G 2.4 million units I.M.</u> *(MIS)
or
Consider alternative Rx _____ *(MIS)
Consider alternative Rx _____ *(MIS).

Physician Consultation. For possible secondary or tertiary disease or if diagnostic uncertainty, treatment failure, or for acute emotional instability.

Referral.

Follow-up Plan. Serologic testing to be repeated: in <u>3</u>, <u>6</u>, and <u>9</u> months for primary, for secondary in <u>12</u> and <u>24</u> months and yearly for the next 5 years. Re-treatment is needed if quantitative serology titers do not decrease four-fold within one year. Re-emphasize the need for follow-up.

	Initials	Date
* unless allergic, contraindicated,	Physician	
or pregnant/lactating	ARNP	

Condyloma Acuminata, Adult Men

EVALUATION/DIAGNOSTIC PROTOCOL

Subjective

History. How were lesions discovered, are there any accompanying symptoms? Obtain sexual and contraceptive history.

Objective

Physical Examination. Complete genital exam (this may need to be done with dilute acetic acid solution). Consider rectal exam.

Lab. If diagnosis in doubt, consider shave biopsy of a single lesion. Consider testing for co-existing STDs, HIV.

Assess severity and extent of disease. **Differential diagnosis** includes condyloma lata, molluscum contagiosum, seborrheic keratosis, and skin neoplasms. **Complications.** Urethral meatal obstruction and transmission to partner(s).

PLAN/MANAGEMENT PROTOCOL

General Measures. Discuss the incubation period, which is variable from 3 weeks to 12 months with 3 months being the average. Discuss modes of transmission and prevention. Strongly recommend routine use of condoms.

Specific Measures. Apply podophyllin 25% solution in tincture of benzoin every week until lesions have disappeared. Do not use for more than 6 weeks without consulting physician. The solution should be applied directly and only to the lesion(s). The patient must be instructed to wash gently with soap and water in 3-9 hours (number of hours depends on level of discomfort and number of hours tolerated after the preceding treatment).

Physician Consultation. Consider for severe disease or if the diagnosis is unclear. Similarly, consider consulting physician if lack of therapeutic response after several applications.

Referral. Consider urologic referral if meatal involvement or extensive disease.

Immediate Transfer. Usually not indicated.

Follow-up Plan. Every week or sooner if signs or symptoms of secondary infection lesion/treatment site develop. Subsequent follow-up as needed for recurrences.

	Initials	Date
* unless allergic, contraindicated, or pregnant/lactating	Physician	
	ARNP	

<u>Herpes Genitalis</u>
<u>Primary and Recurrent</u>
<u>Adult Men</u>

EVALUATION/DIAGNOSTIC PROTOCOL
<u>Subjective</u>
History. Primary symptoms (general malaise, fever, inguinal lymphadenopathy) with vesicles or ulcers on or about the genitalia within a few weeks of sexual contact. Recurrent history may have some of the initial symptomatology and usually a smaller number of lesions and less discomfort.

<u>Objective</u>
Physical Examination. Complete genital examination.

Lab. Viral (herpes) cultures or herpes titers (acute and convalescent) may be indicated. This is particularly true in definitively establishing the diagnosis in a primary occurrence. Consider testing for co-existing STDs, HIV.

<u>Assess</u> severity of the primary infection. **Differential Diagnosis** includes primary syphilis, chancroid, **Complications.** Secondary infection and acute urinary retention, and as relate to social ramifications.

PLAN/MANAGEMENT PROTOCOL
General Measures. For primary or recurrent infection, explain to patient that symptoms last 5-10 days, and that viral shedding after a primary infection may occur for 2-6 weeks. With recurrent, viral shedding is present with prodromal symptoms and until active lesions have healed (average 10 days). Sexual contact should be avoided during these times. Strongly recommend routine use of condoms.

Patients may need counseling for depression and anxiety.

Specific Measures.   PRIMARY OR RECURRENT
Should be treated with oral acyclovir _____*(MIS).

                                RECURRENT
With chronic suppressive therapy with oral acyclovir _____*(MIS)
                                or
with intermittent therapy with oral acyclovir _____*(MIS).
(However, there is no definitive treatment to prevent recurrences.)

Physician Consultation. Consider for severe primary infection or for acute emotional instability.

Referral.

Follow-up Plan. If not considerably improved in _____ days, sooner if worse. If on chronic suppressive therapy, check liver function test every _____ months.

	Initials	Date
* unless allergic, contraindicated, or pregnant/lactating	Physician ARNP	

Condoms

EVALUATION/DIAGNOSTIC PROTOCOL

<u>Subjective</u>

History. Sexual history, motivation and need.

<u>Objective</u>

Physical Examination. Not necessary.

Lab. Not necessary.

<u>Assess</u> appropriateness of method for individual and/or couple. **Complication** is contact allergy (rare).

PLAN/MANAGEMENT PROTOCOL

General Measures. Discuss advantages and benefits of condom use (**latex** for STD prevention as well as birth control method). Teach how to properly use (incorporate into love-making), remove, and store. Advise that contraceptive foam should always be used by female partner for increased effectiveness. Advise to use water-soluble lubricant only, not petroleum jelly. Provide or recommend educational materials. Also refer to most recent <u>Consumer Reports</u> for condom evaluation.

Specific Measures. Advise patient that condoms are relatively inexpensive and available at all drug stores over the counter.

Physician Consultation. Usually not necessary. Consider if patient is infected with HIV and seeking advice on safe sexual practice.

Referral.

Follow-up Plan. Consider individual or couple follow-up visit if birth control method has been difficult issue.

	Initials	Date
* unless allergic, contraindicated,	Physician	
or pregnant/lactating	ARNP	

CHAPTER 9
GYNECOLOGIC

Abnormal Pap Smear

EVALUATION/DIAGNOSTIC PROTOCOL
Subjective
History. GYN history including previous abnormal Paps and treatments of them, symptoms suggestive of gynecologic disease, family history of cancer, sexual history.

Objective
Physical Examination. Genital and rectal inspection, speculum exam, and bimanual pelvic exam as indicated.

Lab. Cervical cultures to detect chlamydia or gonorrhea infections; wet mount slide to detect trichomonas, monilia, or gardnerella. Consider HPV testing. Repeat Pap after treatment or in _____ weeks.

Assess degree of dysplasia and whether inflammatory component is present. **Differential Diagnosis** includes HPV disease (warty atypia, cervical condyloma), severe dysplasia, Ca in situ or invasive Ca, cervicitis. **Complications** relate to advancement of cervical disease.

PLAN/MANAGEMENT PROTOCOL
General Measures. Make every effort to reassure the patient undergoing evaluation. Remember that even those patients likely to have a malignancy have an opportunity for definitive and successful therapy. All abnormal Pap smears require diligent follow-up, whether referral for colposcopy is immediate or pending repeat Pap in 4-6 weeks.

Specific Measures. Treat infections as outlined in appropriate sections depending on causative organism.
Consider Rx _____*(MIS)
                                          or
topical _____*(MIS).

Physician Consultation. Establish criteria for physician consultation on abnormal Pap smears. Of necessity, these must be directed at your laboratory's cytology classification system (e.g., consider consulting on all Class IIs with atypia). Establish colposcopy criteria.

Establish referral criteria.

Referral.

Immediate Transfer. None.

Follow-up Plan. For diagnosis of infection if indicated, then repeat Pap in _____. Again, consider colposcopy.

	Initials	Date
Physician		
ARNP		

* unless allergic, contraindicated, or pregnant/lactating

<u>Pregnant, First Trimester or</u>
<u>Pregnant, the First Visit</u>

EVALUATION/DIAGNOSTIC PROTOCOL

Subjective

History. Conduct the history in a nonjudgmental manner. Last normal menses and interval menstrual history, previous normal menses, and past menstrual history. Ovulatory history if known. Was the patient trying to conceive? Obstetrical history (pregnancies, children [living, gestation, delivery, labor course, complication, APGARs, birth weight], spontaneous miscarriages, therapeutic abortions). General medical history (recent or current illnesses and treatments). Past medical history. Family history (average gestations of sisters, mother, maternal aunts and grandmothers). Social history (current living circumstances, occupational exposures, etc.). Father's history. Review of systems (nutritional history [ideal body weight, dietary practices]), unhealthy habits [caffeine, tobacco, alcohol and illicit drug use], complete systems review.

Objective

Physical Examination. Vital signs, general appearance, HEENT, neck (thyroid), chest, breasts, lungs, cardiovascular, abdominal, pelvic (fundal height, adnexa, pelvic measurements, include PAP, and STD screens), rectal, back and extremities, skin, neurologic.

Lab. In addition to those done during pelvic, CBC, type Rh and antibody screen, serology, Rubella titer, urinalysis (screening culture), fasting blood sugar. Consider hepatitis screen, HIV, hemoglobin electrophoresis. Consider sonography, quantitative serum HCG and alpha-fetoprotein and other tests for fetal assessment.

Assessment in pure medical terms is directed at determining whether this is a viable IUP, the gestational age, and the maternal and fetal risks and prognosis. **Differential Diagnosis** is directed at determining there is a viable IUP **Complications.** The complications of pregnancy at its various stages and in various circumstances are well known and numerous. The authors recommend a standard obstetrical text, consider <u>Ambulatory Obsterics: Protocols for Nurse Practitioners</u> by Star, W.L. et al., University of California.

PLAN/MANAGEMENT PROTOCOL

General Measures. Discuss your findings and expectations. Review the prenatal care plans and discuss the tests ordered and planned. Preferably provide a writtten schedule. Explain the physiology of pregnancy and attendant changes. Discuss diet, exercise and hygiene, and provide educational materials (see <u>The First Trimester</u> instruction sheet).

Specific Measures.
Consider prenatal vitamins_____*(MIS).

Physician Consultation. Establish criteria.

Referral. Establish criteria for obstetrical referral or termination referral.

Immediate Transfer. Establish criteria.

Follow-up Plan. Establish criteria.

	Initials	Date
* unless allergic, contraindicated, or pregnant/lactating	Physician ARNP	

Fibrocystic Breasts

EVALUATION/DIAGNOSTIC PROTOCOL
Subjective
History. Medical, gynecologic and obstetrical. Previous personal or family history. Current medications OTC/Rx/Illicit. Current habit history (caffeine consumption, chocolate, and tobacco). Patient's perception of the problem and concerns. L.M.P.

Objective
Physical Examination. General appearance, vital signs, thorough breast exam (consider using a breast grid diagramming system).

Lab. If age and or risk factor appropriate, then consider mammography.

Assess the severity of the disease both in anatomic terms but also as to the degree of patient discomfort. **Differential Diagnosis**. Must always be distinguished form breast carcinoma. **Complications**. Usually just as relates to degree of discomfort. Patient's with this sometimes are at higher risk for breast cancer. They do, however, have greater difficulty with self-examination, which is stressful.

PLAN/MANAGEMENT PROTOCOL
General Measures. Explain to patients that this is mainly a benign problem Its symptoms can diminish with habit modification, particularly drastic reduction in caffeine and nicotine intake (be absolute about the need to quit smoking). Similarly, weight reduction helps the overweight woman.

Breast self-examination is critically important. Provide teaching model or video. Provide or recommend other educational material (such as Dr. Susan Love's Breast Book by Consumer Reports). Reinforce this at every examination.

Specific Measures.
Consider for symptomatic relief an Rx for _____ *(MIS).

Also consider _____ *(MIS).

Physician Consultation. Consider for severe breast involvement or if dominant mass(es) (see New Breast Mass).

Referral.

Immediate Transfer.

Follow-up Plan. Involves re-examining in _____ weeks and thereafter every _____ months.

	Initials	Date
Physician		
ARNP		

* unless allergic, contraindicated, or pregnant/lactating

New Breast Mass

EVALUATION/DIAGNOSTIC PROTOCOL

Subjective

History. Breast history as part of gynecologic and obstetrical history. Previous masses and course. When was this first noticed? Has it changed? Are there accompanying symptoms? Current medications OTC/Rx/Illicit. Current habits. Detailed family history of all cancers and particularly of the breast.

Objective

Physical Examination. General appearance, vital signs and thorough breast exam include chest wall and axilla (consider using a breast grid diagramming system).

Lab. Mammography and, if needed, ultrasound. Consider needle aspiration, needle biopsy, or excision biopsy by consultant (even if negative mammography which has an error rate of 10-15%).

Assess probability of the mass being malignant. If any suspicion pursue definitive diagnosis. **Differential Diagnosis** includes benign causes such as cysts and fibroadenomas(over 4 out of 5 biopsies are benign); less common are the malignancies (yet 1 in 9 women develop malignancy). **Complications** relate to the tissue diagnosis if this is a malignancy. Even during the diagnostic process patients are very anxious.

PLAN/MANAGEMENT PROTOCOL

General Measures. Make every effort to reassure the patient undergoing evaluation. Similarly remember that even those patients likely to have a malignancy have opportunity for definitive and successful therapy. Explain to patients that this is usually a benign problem. Symptoms of benign masses can diminish with habit modification, particularly drastic reduction in caffeine and nicotine intake (be absolute about the need to quit smoking). Similarly, weight reduction helps the overweight woman.

    Breast self-examination is critically important. Provide teaching model or video. Provide or recommend other educational material (such as Dr. Susan Love's Breast Book by Consumer Reports). Reinforce this at every examination.

Specific Measures. For a soft, mobile, mass in a low risk patient, consider re-examination in _____ weeks.

Physician Consultation. For a suspicious mass or any in a high risk patient, opt for definitive diagnosis.

Referral. To surgeon as recommended by physician.

Follow-up Plan. Recheck or refer soon after mammography.

Initials   Date

* unless allergic, contraindicated,   Physician
or pregnant/lactating   ARNP

Mastitis

EVALUATION/DIAGNOSTIC PROTOCOL

Subjective

History. Onset and course. Obstetrical and gynecologic history, general medical history. Previous personal history. Current medications prescription, over the counter, illicit. Current habit history (caffeine, alcohol, foods). Nursing history and practices.

Objective

Physical Examination. General appearance, vital signs, thorough breast exam (nipple fissures or abrasions, lobular or generalized involvement with erythema, distention, "caking," even induration).

Lab. If age and risk factors appropriate consider mammography (discuss with radiologist the optimal circumstance for the study to be done if nursing). Consider culture of nipple discharge. Consider prolactin in the non-nursing or not recently nursing.

Assess severity. **Differential Diagnosis**. Breast abscess, squamous metaplasia of the ducts (Zuzka's disease), duct ectasia, and even thrombophlebitis (Mondor's disease). **Complications**.

PLAN/MANAGEMENT PROTOCOL

General Measures. Reassure the nursing mother that nursing can and should be continued (even with antibiotic use), preferably nursing the involved breast first (pumping may be a suitable alternative). Apply moist heat which can often be done in hot shower (also a good place to manipulate the "caked" breast).

Specific Measures

Consider antibiotic therapy _____ *(MIS)

Consider analgesic therapy _____ *(MIS)

Physician Consultation. Consider depending on severity or lack of subsequent therapeutic response.

Referral.

Immediate Transfer. For sepsis.

Follow-up Plan. _____ days/weeks, sooner if no improvement in _____ days and sooner if worsening.

Initials   Date

* unless allergic, contraindicated,   Physician
or pregnant/lactating   ARNP

Premenstrual Syndrome

EVALUATION/DIAGNOSTIC PROTOCOL
Subjective
History. Thorough history of symptoms that is retrospective, unstructured, and details timing of symptom(s) in relation to menstrual cycle. GYN history, past medical history, family history, and drug history.

Objective
Physical Examination. Complete physical exam usually indicated.

Lab. Consider CBC and thyroid survey, including TSH.

Assess to determine severity and type of syndrome. **Differential Diagnosis** includes dysmenorrhea, endometriosis, psychiatric disorders, anemia, and thyroid disease. **Complications.** Psychologic decompensation which has personal, family, occupational and social ramifications.

PLAN/MANAGEMENT PROTOCOL
General Measures. In most cases, intervention should be withheld until an accurate chart of symptoms with timing during cycle is kept for three months. This will establish the diagnosis and guide treatment. Practitioner should recognize importance of placebo effect in relieving symptoms. Educate patient and family about nature of etiology to foster supportive environment. Regular exercise and small frequent meals high in complex carbohydrates and low in salt and sugar may help. Beware of potential for alcohol use and dependency. Consider referral to local support group or tell patient about supportive bi-monthly newsletter, Cycles, P.O. Box 524, Sharon, ME 02067.

Specific Measures. Rx treatment usually aimed at suppressing cyclic ovarian activity.
With consultation, consider _____ *(MIS)
                                          or
_____ *(MIS).

Consider symptomatic therapy _____ *(MIS).

Physician Consultation. Consider if having difficulty establishing diagnosis, before any drug intervention is instituted or if psychiatric component is significant.

Referral. May be helpful or necessary for professional counseling. If therapeutic approach not successful, consider gynecologic or gyne-endocrinologic evaluation.

Immediate Transfer.

Follow-up Plan. In _____ months to review patient's symptom chart, then every _____ months and PRN for problems.

	Initials	Date
* unless allergic, contraindicated, or pregnant/lactating	Physician ARNP	

Dysmenorrhea

EVALUATION/DIAGNOSTIC PROTOCOL
Subjective
History. Onset and progression of symptoms, aggravating and alleviating factors, associated symptoms, past medical history with attention to GYN history.

Objective
Physical Examination. General appearance, vital signs, abdominal and pelvic exam.

Lab. Pap smear and cervical cultures as indicated, UA, CBC or ultrasound as indicated on presentation.

Assess if this is primary dysmenorrhea or due to underlying pathology. Assess severity of pain and success with patient's previous attempts to deal with it. **Differential Diagnosis** relates to underlying pathology such as endometriosis, uterine fibroids, P.I.D., ovarian cysts, or masses. UTI or appendicitis may be cause for sudden onset or exacerbation. **Complications.** Severe pain inhibiting normal functioning.

PLAN/MANAGEMENT PROTOCOL
General Measures. Counseling patient that there is physical cause of pain and that it is not psychological. Reassure patient that no pelvic disease has been found and that symptoms will not be life-long. Advise regular physical exercise and teach pelvic/back relaxation exercises. Recommend hot bath, application of heating pad, and/or gentle massage. Although alcohol can relieve symptoms, be aware of potential for dependency.

Specific Measures. Therapy is directed at inhibiting prostaglandins with PGSIs
Rx _____ or _____*(MIS)
or
_____*(MIS).

Consider OC use when appropriate _____*(MIS).

Physician Consultation. Consider for secondary dysmenorrhea or primary cases not responding to therapy.

Referral.

Immediate Transfer. Usually not necessary.

Follow-up Plan. For routine GYN care or as needed.

Initials   Date

* unless allergic, contraindicated,   Physician
or pregnant/lactating   ARNP

Endometriosis

EVALUATION/DIAGNOSTIC PROTOCOL
<u>Subjective</u>.
History. Onset of symptoms, description of pain (time of cycle, how long into menses does it last, worsening over time, rectal pressure). Complete GYN history; note problems with infertility, dyspareunia. Menopausal? (Rarely seen after menopause.)

<u>Objective</u>
Physical Examination. Abdominal and pelvic exam, including rectovaginal exam. (classic finding is tender utero-sacral ligaments with fixed uterine retroversion). Note tenderness or adnexal masses (ovarian choclate cyst).

Lab. Consider _____.

Differential Diagnosis. Primary dysmenorrhea, secondary dysmenorrhea, pelvic inflammatory disease, other causes of pelvic mass. **Complications.** Gastrointestinal involvement, infertility, disabling symptoms, rupture of ovarian endometrioma causing peritonitis.

PLAN/MANAGEMENT PROTOCOL
General Measures. Explain disease process (including need to keep diary of symptoms for at least a few months). Explain need for laparoscopy for definitive diagnosis. Treatment depends on age, severity of symptoms, staging of disease and desire for fertility. Aerobic exercise may improve symptoms by raising the estrone-estradiol ratio. Pregnancy will significantly improve condition.

Specific Measures.
Consider for mild disease symptomatic treatment.

Consider NSAID _____ *(MIS)
and/or
oral contraceptive _____ *(MIS).

Consider more definitive Rx with consultation or previous established criteria.

Physician Consultation. Consider with diagnostic uncertainty or if needing referral to gynecologist.

Referral. To gynecologist _____ for laparoscopy and management as indicated.

Follow-up Plan. Depends on whether patient is being followed by gynecologist. If you are managing mild disease consider every _____ months, or as necessary to promote patient's understanding, general good health and comfort.

		Initials	Date
* unless allergic, contraindicated, or pregnant/lactating	Physician ARNP		

Uterine Leiomyomas (Fibroids) &
Adenomyosis

EVALUATION/DIAGNOSTIC PROTOCOL

Subjective

History. Complete gynecologic and obstetric history with attention too onset and course of dysmenorrhea, pelvic pain or pressure, changes in uterine bleeding. General medical history, family history, social history, review of systems. What does the patient think is wrong?

Objective

Physical Examination. Vital signs, general appearance, thyroid, chest, cardio-vascular, abdomen, pelvic and rectal exam.

Lab. Urinalysis, Pap smear, STD screenings, Hct. Consider a pregnancy test. Consider ultrasound of pelvis. Consider CA125.

Assessment. **Differential Diagnosis** includes ovarian tumors, endometriosis, pregnancy (intrauterine or extrauterine), uterine malignacy, abscess, bowel tumors or abscesses. **Complications** include degeneration, infection, severe bleeding and the rare leiomyosarcoma (0.2% of patients).

PLAN/MANAGEMENT PROTOCOL

General Measures. Explain to the patient that this represents an over growth of cells of the uterine wall. When diffuse this is called adenomyosis, but when discreet areas are involved the resultant tumors are also called fibroids. Usually the occurance is not singular. Unless there are signs or symptoms of complications, these can be treated expectantly. Patients must be alerted to the possibility that these can complicate pregnancy and an obstetrical consult should be planned before conceiving.

Specific Measures. There is no satisfactory medical therapy. Surgical therapy is sometimes indicated that decision must be individualized.

Physician Consultation. Consider for newly diagnosed and as needed for changing signs and symptoms.

Referral. To gynecologist _____ when indicated.

Immediate Transfer. For severe hemorrhage, acute abdomen.

Follow-up Plan. Every _____ months and as needed for symptom change.

	Initials	Date
* unless allergic, contraindicated, or pregnant/lactating	Physician ARNP	

Secondary Amenorrhea

EVALUATION/DIAGNOSTIC PROTOCOL
Subjective
History. Menstrual history, birth control method used if indicated, diet and exercise history, emotional state, history of galactorrhea, drug history, other associated symptoms.

Objective
Physical Examination. Weight, vital signs, skin exam, breast exam--check for nipple discharge--pelvic exam, complete P/E if indicated.

Lab. Serum HCG as indicated, prolactin and thyroid survey if amenorrhea is present 6 months or more. Consider FSH, LH, and pelvic ultrasound.

Assessment. Primary versus secondary amenorrhea. **Differential Diagnosis** includes pregnancy, thyroid disease, pituitary tumors, systemic illness, polycystic ovarian disease, psychotropic drug use, starvation dieting, adrenal disease. **Complications** include endometrial hyperplasia and osteoporosis.

PLAN/MANAGEMENT PROTOCOL
General Measures. If diagnosis is functional amenorrhea, usually re-establishment of menstrual cycles is spontaneous. Counsel patient to eat balanced meals and assist with stress-coping strategies. Change in vigorous exercise program may be indicated.

Specific Measures. If pregnancy is ruled out, trial of progesterone to induce menstrual shedding is usually indicated.
Rx _____*(MIS)
                                                 and
if menses is induced, may begin Rx _____*(MIS)
                                          or
alternative Rx _____*(MIS)
to induce normal cycles and prevent complications of amenorrhea.

Physician Consultation. Consider for amenorrhea of more than 6 months and whenever a work-up beyond pregnancy test is indicated.

Referral. Pending physician consultation to gynecologist or endocrinologist as indicated by preliminary evaluation. Professional mental health counseling as indicated.

Immediate Transfer. None.

Follow-up Plan. Initially every _____ month(s) until diagnosis is established, then as needed.

	Initials	Date
* unless allergic, contraindicated,	Physician	
or pregnant/lactating	ARNP	

Acute Cystitis, Women

EVALUATION/DIAGNOSTIC PROTOCOL
Subjective
History. General, genitourinary review of symptoms, course potentiating factors and precipitating events. Be certain to obtain contraceptive method history.

Objective
Physical Examination. General appearance, vital signs, abdominal and pelvic exam.

Lab. Urinalysis, culture and consider sensitivities.

Assess accuracy of diagnostic testing and contribution of complicating factors (anatomic, neoplastic, physiologic/mechanical dysfunction, presence of other STDs). **Differential Diagnosis** is among other urinary or genital tract infections. **Complications**. Chronic infections, which can be problematic in pregnancy.

PLAN/MANAGEMENT PROTOCOL
General Measures. Encourage patients to force fluids and in the future to consider urinating frequently, making an effort to completely empty the bladder. Review female hygiene, avoiding or limiting douching, feminine hygiene sprays, deodorized tampons. Remind patients they may benefit from cotton crotched underwear.
 If infection related to sexual intercourse, recommend urinating before and after. (If diaphragm use a contributing factor than consider a change in methods). If needed, recommend water soluble lubricant.

Specific Measures.
Consider standard antibiotic regime, Rx _____*(MIS)
                                              or
alternative standard Rx _____*(MIS)
                                              or
consider single dose antibiotic Rx _____*(MIS).

Some patients benefit from Rx for urinary tract analgesic dye _____*(MIS).

Physician Consultation. Consider for severe pain, retention, evidence of bacteremia. Similarly consult for recurrences or treatment failure.

Referral.

Immediate Transfer. Should be considered for toxicity or severe retention.

Follow-up Plan. In _____ days, sooner if worse, or if desired therapeutic response not achieved in _____ days. Follow-up urine culture _____ days after antibiotic therapy completed.

                                                        Initials   Date
* unless allergic, contraindicated,   Physician
or pregnant/lactating   ARNP

Pyelonephritis, Women

EVALUATION/DIAGNOSTIC PROTOCOL
Subjective
History. General, urinary, review of symptoms, course, potentiating factors and precipitating events. Be certain to obtain date of last menstrual period and contraceptive method history.

Objective
Physical Examination. General appearance, vital signs, abdominal and pelvic exam.

Lab. Urinalysis and culture (single type colony counts of as little as 1,000 per milliliter may be significant). Consider sensitivities.

Assess severity and in particular evidence of septicemia. **Differential Diagnosis** includes other urinary tract infections (see Cystitis, Women and Nephrolithiasis, Adults). **Complications.** Chronic infection and renal damage.

PLAN/MANAGEMENT PROTOCOL
General Measures. Encourage patients to force fluids and in the future to consider urinating frequently, making an effort to completely empty the bladder.

Review female hygiene measures. If infection related to sexual intercourse, recommend urinating before and after.

Specific Measures.
Consider oral antibiotic Rx _____*(MIS)
or
alternative antibiotic regime _____*(MIS).

Physician Consultation. For severe infection or toxic appearing patient, significant underlying factors or severe pain. Similarly, consult for recurrences.

Referral. Pending physician consultation to urologist _____.

Immediate Transfer. For toxic or unstable patient to _____.

Follow-up Plan. In _____ day(s), sooner if worse, or if desired therapeutic response not achieved in _____ days. Follow-up urinalysis or culture in _____ day(s). After cessation of treatment, consider serial urine cultures.

		Initials	Date
* unless allergic, contraindicated,	Physician		
or pregnant/lactating	ARNP		

Candidal Vulvovaginitis

EVALUATION/DIAGNOSTIC PROTOCOL
Subjective
History. Symptoms, course, predisposing factors (recent antibiotic usage), predisposing/underlying conditions, last menstrual period and current contraceptive measures.

Objective
Physical Examination. General appearance, vital signs, pelvic exam.

Lab. KOH smear and/or candidal culture.

Assess severity. **Differential Diagnosis** is among the other vaginal infection and remember that mixed vaginitis is a common occurrence. **Complications.** Persistent or recurrent infection, dyspareunia.

PLAN/MANAGEMENT PROTOCOL
General Measures. Explain the general benignity of this infection. Review female hygiene and diet (consider cutting intake of simple carbohydrate). Wear loose-fitting underclothes and clothes, at least cotton crotched underwear.

Specific Measures.
Give Rx for antifungal vaginal cream and/or suppository _____*(MIS)

and/or

alternative Rx _____*(MIS).

Consider vinegar water douching (2 tablespoons of vinegar/quart of lukewarm water).

For frequent recurrences, consider oral antifungal Rx (to eradicate gastrointestinal reservoir) _____*(MIS).
Also consider examining and treating her paramour.

Physician Consultation. Consider for severe or repeated infections. Consider evaluating patient for diabetes.

Referral.

Immediate Transfer.

Follow-up Plan. Consider follow-up in _____ days, sooner if worse or if symptoms persist, then re-examine in _____ weeks.

Initials   Date

* unless allergic, contraindicated,   Physician
or pregnant/lactating   ARNP

Trichomonas Vaginitis

EVALUATION/DIAGNOSTIC PROTOCOL
<u>Subjective</u>
History. General history, urinary and genital/sexual history, onset of symptoms, and course. Patient's own description of discharge, any vaginal symptomatology (soreness, itching, dyspareunia, or postcoital spotting), other accompanying symptomatology, previous history of STDs, last menstrual period and current contraceptive methodology.

<u>Objective</u>
Physical Examination. General appearance, vital signs, abdomen, and complete pelvic exam (frothy green classic discharge may actually vary in appearance and consistency).

Lab. Wet prep. Consider testing for other STDs, HIV.

<u>Assess</u> severity. **Differential Diagnosis** includes other vaginal infections (see <u>Candida Vaginitis</u> and <u>Gardnerella Vaginitis</u>). **Complications.** None.

PLAN/MANAGEMENT PROTOCOL
General Measures. Explain that this is often a sexually transmitted protozoa, but that it can be spread by other mechanisms, from wet bathing suits and washcloths to douche nozzles. Remind a patient in a stable relationship that the organism can be harbored in the vagina for decades without being symptomatic. Sympathetic counseling can prevent social trauma. Strongly recommend routine use of condoms.

Specific Measures.
Treat with oral Rx, short course _____ *(MIS)

(be cautious about retreatment frequency)   or

Oral Rx, long course _____ *(MIS).
Remember to treat partner(s).
If pregnant, then treat topically _____ *(MIS).

Physician Consultation. Consider if patient is not satisfied with explanation. Also, consult if refractory to therapy.

Referral.

Follow-up Plan. Consider recheck in _____ weeks, sooner if recurrent or worse.

                                                    Initials   Date

* unless allergic, contraindicated,   Physician
or pregnant/lactating   ARNP

Gardnerella Vaginitis

EVALUATION/DIAGNOSTIC PROTOCOL

Subjective

History. General history, urinary and genital/sexual history, onset of symptoms and course. Patient's own description of discharge, any vaginal symptomatology (soreness, itching, dyspareunia, or postcoital spotting), other accompanying symptoms, previous history of STDs, last menstrual period and current contraceptive methods.

Objective

Physical Examination. General appearance, vital signs, abdomen and complete pelvic exam (thin malodorous greyish-white discharge).

Lab. Wet prep shows typical "clue" cells. Consider testing for other STD's, HIV.

Assess severity. **Differential Diagnosis** includes the other vaginal infections (see Trichomonas Vaginitis and consider Chlamydia). **Complications**. Recurrence or persistence.

PLAN/MANAGEMENT PROTOCOL

General Measures. Explain that this is often a sexually transmitted disease but commonly may be considered part of the normal vaginal microbrial flora. This ability for the gardnerella bacterial to remain in a sort of ecological balance indefinitely before creating sypmtoms can confuse the issue of when it may have been transmitted. Partner will require treatment. Strong recommend routine use of condoms.

Specific Measures.
Treat with oral Rx for metronidazole _____*(MIS)
(be cautious about retreatment frequency)
As an alternative, consider Rx _____*(MIS).

Physician Consultation. Consider for severe infection or treatment failure or if patient is not satisfied with explanation.

Referral.

Follow-up Plan. If symptoms recur.

	Initials	Date
* unless allergic, contraindicated, or pregnant/lactating	Physician ARNP	

Chlamydia, Adult Women

EVALUATION/DIAGNOSTIC PROTOCOL

Subjective

History. Onset and course, possible exposure, last menstrual period, contraceptive methodology.

Objective

Physical Examination. General appearance, vital signs, pelvic and rectal.

Lab. Endocervical chlamydial culture or prep, and consider similar rectal test. Consider testing for other STD's, HIV.

Assess severity. **Differential Diagnosis.** The presence or absence of other STDs, non-infectious cervicitis. **Complications** are progression to pelvic inflammatory disease and the attendant complications. Social ramifications may be complex and disturbing. Newborns can be infected at delivery.

PLAN/MANAGEMENT PROTOCOL

General Measures. Remind patient this infection, though asymptomatic, will not resolve without treatment. Emphasize the need for follow-up culture.

Patient and partners should refrain from sexual activity until they have completed simultaneous treatment. Strongly recommend routine use of condoms to protect against STDs.

Specific Measures.

Rx for oral tetracycline antibiotic _____ *(MIS)

or

alternative antibiotic Rx _____ *(MIS).

Physician Consultation. Consider for severe infection/possible PID, treatment failure or frequent recurrence, and especially for pregnant or lactating patients.

Referral.

Immediate Transfer. For severe pelvic inflammatory disease.

Follow-up Plan. Follow-up and re-culture in _____ weeks, sooner if worse.

Initials   Date

* unless allergic, contraindicated,   Physician
or pregnant/lactating   ARNP

Condyloma Acuminata, Women

EVALUATION/DIAGNOSTIC PROTOCOL

<u>Subjective</u>

History. How were the lesions discovered? Are there any accompanying symptoms? Obtain sexual and contraceptive history.

<u>Objective</u>

Physical Examination. Complete pelvic examination with Pap smear. Consider rectal exam. Weak acetic acid solution can assist in identification of lesions. Consider using magnification (colposcopy if ARNP qualified).

Lab. Pap smear. If diagnosis is in doubt, consider shaved biopsy of a single lesion. Consider HPV testing and consider HPV typing. Consider testing for other STDs, HIV.

<u>Assess</u> severity and extent of disease. **Differential Diagnosis** includes other vulva lesions. **Complications** reflects the measures used to remove them. Most significant is the association with cervical cancer. Also, these can cause significant complications in pregnancy. Social ramifications.

PLAN/MANAGEMENT PROTOCOL

General Measures. Discuss the incubation period, which is variable from 3 weeks to 12 months (with 3 months being the average). Discuss modes of transmission and prevention. Emphasize the need to have contacts examined. Sympathetic counseling can assist the patient in coping with this frustrating condition. Strongly recommend routine use of condoms to protect against STDs. Explain the association with cervical cancer and emphatically recommend Pap smears every _____ months.

Patients may need counseling for depression and anxiety. Often it is helpful to discuss more about this infection at subsequent visits when the patients are likely to be less upset and better able to absorb the information.

Specific Measures.
Treat vulva lesions by _____(PIS or *MIS).

Authors realize that some ARNPs may be qualified to:
Treat vaginal lesions by _____(PIS or *MIS).
Treat cervical lesions by _____(PIS os *MIS).
otherwise the physician should be consulted or these should be referred.

Physician Consultation. Consider for widespread or severe disease, and in particular if the diagnosis is unclear. Similarly, consult physician if there a lack of therapeutic response.

Referral.

Immediate Transfer.

Follow-up Plan. Re-examination and/or re-treat every _____ week(s)/month(s) or as indicated. Follow-up Pap smears every _____ month(s).

                                             Initials   Date

* unless allergic, contraindicated,   Physician
or pregnant/lactating   ARNP

<u>Herpes Genitalis</u>
<u>Primary and Recurrent</u>
<u>Adult Women</u>

EVALUATION/DIAGNOSTIC PROTOCOL
<u>Subjective</u>
History. Primary symptoms (general malaise, fever, inguinal lymphadenopathy) with vesicles or ulcers on or about the genitalia within a few weeks of sexual contact. Recurrent history may have some of the initial symptomatology and usually a smaller number of lesions and less discomfort.

<u>Objective</u>
Physical Examination. Complete pelvic examination.

Lab. Viral (herpes) cultures or herpes titers (acute and convalescent) may be indicated. This is particularly true in definitively establishing the diagnosis in a primary occurrence. Consider testing for other STDs, HIV.

<u>Assess</u> severity of primary infection, or frequency and severity of recurrences. **Differential Diagnosis.** Primary syphilis, chancroids, vulvar abrasions, excoriations (secondary to candida or other dermatitidies). **Complications** are significant as an infected mother can transmit the virus to her infant at birth. Social ramifications.

PLAN/MANAGEMENT PROTOCOL
General Measures. Explain that this is often a sexually transmitted disease. For primary or recurrent infection, explain to patient that symptoms last 5-10 days, and that viral shedding after a primary infection may occur for 2-6 weeks. With recurrent, viral shedding is present with prodromal symptoms and until active lesions have healed (average 10 days). Sexual contact should be avoided during these times. Strongly recommend routine use of condoms to prevent STDs.
      Recommend Pap smears every _____ months.
      Patients may need counseling for depression and anxiety. Often it is helpful to discuss more about this infection at subsequent visits when the patients are likely to be less upset and better able to absorb the information.

Specific Measures. Primary or recurrent should be treated with oral acyclovir _____*(MIS). Recurrent disease can be treated either with chronic suppressive therapy with oral acyclovir _____*(MIS) or with intermittent therapy with oral acyclovir _____*(MIS). (However, there is no definitive treatment to prevent recurrences.)

Physician Consultation. Consider for severe primary infection or for acute emotional instability.

Referral.

Immediate Transfer.

Follow-up Plan. Consider recheck in _____ days to assess therapeutic response and emotional state of patient. Otherwise, if not considerably improved in _____ days, sooner if worse. If on suppressive therapy, check every _____ month(s), CBC and liver function tests.

					Initials	Date
* unless allergic, contraindicated, or pregnant/lactating

Physician
ARNP

Gonorrhea

EVALUATION/DIAGNOSTIC PROTOCOL
Subjective
History. Description of symptoms; known contact to someone with gonorrhea, coexistent STDs. (Consider pharyngeal, urethral, cervical, or anorectal sites of infection.) Note: incubation period, 3-14 days. 10% of males and 75% of females are asymptomatic.

Objective
Physical Examination. As indicated by sexual history.

Lab. Females: Thayer-Martin culture of endocervical canal and other sites as indicated. Other tests to rule out co-existing STDs.

Assess severity of disease. **Differential diagnosis.** Known gonococcal urethritis, trichomonal urethritis, UTI, vaginitis, cervicitis due to Chlamydia or other infections. **Complications.** Pelvic inflammatory disease and ultimately sterility.

PLAN/MANAGEMENT PROTOCOL
General Measures. Treat all patients with positive gram stain or cultures as well as all patients with known contact to someone with gonorrhea. Patient education re: nature of disease and outcome, abstinence until follow-up culture is negative, importance of notifying partner(s), and prevention. Recommend use of latex condoms. Report cases to Public Health Department.

Specific Measures. Drug of choice is <u>Ceftriaxone, 125-250 mg IM once</u> *(MIS)
or
_____*(MIS)
or
_____*(MIS)
followed by _____*(MIS)
or
_____*(MIS).

Physician Consultation. Consider for severe pelvic inflammatory disease. In a child diagnosed with gonorrhea, always consult and proceed as if it were a case of sexual abuse. Consider for repeated treatment failures or if there are any other systemic manifestations.

Referral. Consider treating severe PID in the hospital.

Immediate Transfer. Usually not necessary.

Follow-up Plan. Repeat culture in _____ days. Emphasize abstinence until negative culture is obtained.

                                                          Initials   Date

* unless allergic, contraindicated,   Physician
or pregnant/lactating   ARNP

Syphilis, Women

EVALUATION/DIAGNOSTIC PROTOCOL
Subjective
History. Description of symptoms: known exposure to syphilis, sexual and contraceptive history. Note: primary stage--incubation period, 9-90 days; secondary stage--3-8 weeks after chancre is healed, disappears spontaneously in 2-6 weeks; latent stage--patient remains asymptomatic; tertiary stage--10-20 years after initial exposure.

Objective/Physical Examination. Genital exam or as indicated by history.

Lab. Dark field microscopic exam if available. VDRL/RPR, confirm with FTA/ABS (fluorescent treponemal antibody absorption test). Tests for coexisting STDs.

Assess stage of disease and determine the presence of other STDs to ensure treatment of all contacts. Differential Diagnosis includes other STDs and other causes of skin ulcers, including herpes and chancroid. Secondary lues a macular papular dermatitis that is intermittently symptomatic and has a large differential diagnosis (mononucleosis, pityriasis rosea, and the coxsackie viruses). Complications. Cardiovascular disease, central nervous system damage including blindness, congenital infection of the neonate.

PLAN/MANAGEMENT PROTOCOL
General Measures. Patient education concerning disease course and outcome, importance of notifying sexual contacts, need for abstinence until after appropriate treatment, prevention. Report to Public Health Department. Recommend condoms to protect against other STDs.

Specific Measures. Primary, secondary, or latent of less than 1 year. Drug of choice is Penicillin G. Benzathine, 2.4 million units IM once.

Alternatives: _____ *(MIS)
                            or
_____ *(MIS)
                            or
_____ *(MIS).

Continued drug treatment, latent of more than one year duration: drug of choice Penicillin G. Benzathine, 2.4 million units weekly times 3 weeks
                            or
_____ *(MIS)
                            or
_____ *(MIS).

Physician Consultation. Consider if there is diagnostic uncertainty or a treatment failure. Consider if patient is exhibiting signs of tertiary infection. Consult for syphilis in a pregnant women or child or suspected congenital infection in newborn, unless other protocols established.

Referral.

Follow-up Plan. Public Health Department usually will notify patient's contacts. Blood serological testing for primary infection to be repeated in _3_, _6_, and _9_ months. Secondary: repeat in _12_ and _24_ months. Should be non-reactive within 2 years. Early and latent: repeat 2 year for 5 years. 75% of early latent will be non-reactive; 75% of late latent will be reactive more than 5 years. Re-treatment needed if quantitative serology titers do not decrease at least four-fold within 1 year.

* unless allergic, contraindicated,   Physician
or pregnant/lactating   ARNP

Initials   Date

Oral Contraception, Initial Visit

EVALUATION/DIAGNOSTIC PROTOCOL
Subjective
History. Complete past medical history to determine if contraindications are present; family history; sexual history.

Objective
Physical Examination. Vital signs, weight, pelvic and breast exam, including Pap smear if not done within last 6 months. Thyroid, lungs, heart, and abdominal exam unless done within last 6 months.

Lab. Pap smear, test for sexually transmitted diseases when indicated, consider FBS, lipid profile if appropriate, and/or _____.

Assessment. Determine suitability of method for individual's need and presence or absence of contraindications. **Complications** include thromboembolic disease, M.I., phlebitis, hypertension (the risks in the preceding are greatly increased by smokers over 30), liver tumors, myoma, predisposition to gall bladder disease, metabolic and endocrinologic effects.

PLAN/MANAGEMENT PROTOCOL
General Measures. Comprehensive patient education, including how OCs work to prevent pregnancy, proper method of taking, possible side effects and health risks and what to do if problems occur. Review appropriate starting method and provide reinforcing educational materials. Provide patient education materials to reinforce information you have told them. Emphasize and re-emphasize **safe sex practices** and educate about the use of condoms. Consider multi-vitamin and/or vitamin B6 supplementation.

Specific Measures. Low dose, tri-phasic or straight dose combination. Pill choices include: _____*(MIS)
                                                         or
_____*(MIS).

Physician Consultation. Consider for anyone who has relative or possible contraindications. Consider for problematic side effects, including if patient is amenorrheic. Consult if patient becomes pregnant while on OCs.

Referral.

Immediate Transfer.

Follow-up Plan. Check weight and blood pressure and assess side effects in _____ to _____ months, then _____. If over 35, consider lipid profile in _____ months, family history of diabetes consider FBS in _____ months, if BP is borderline elevated, recheck in _____ months. Time follow-up visit with need for next Pap smear and limit refills to that time.

	Initials	Date
* unless allergic, contraindicated,	Physician	
or pregnant/lactating	ARNP	

Oral Contraception, Follow-Up Visit

EVALUATION/DIAGNOSTIC PROTOCOL

Subjective

History. Problems, side effects (especially headaches and visual problems).

Objective

Physical Examination. Vital signs, complete pelvic exam, breast exam, thyroid, lungs, heart, and abdominal exam.

Lab. Pap smear, check for sexually transmitted diseases if indicated. FBS or lipid profile if indicated.

Assess suitability of method for patient.

PLAN/MANAGEMENT PROTOCOL

General Measures. Review how patient is taking pills, severity if side effects are present, and satisfaction of method. Provide additional patient education materials to reinforce information you have told them. Emphasize and re-emphasize **safe sex practices** and educate about the use of condoms.

Specific Measures. Renew OCs for _____ months. Make changes in prescription as indicated.

Physician Consultation. Consider for any serious or "perceived serious" side effects, if previous change in type of OC does not improve patient's symptoms, if patient has developed any relative contraindications.

Referral.

Immediate Transfer. Same as for initial visit.

Follow-up Plan. See initial oral contraceptive section.

Initials   Date

* unless allergic, contraindicated,   Physician
or pregnant/lactating   ARNP

Diaphragm

EVALUATION/DIAGNOSTIC PROTOCOL
<u>Subjective</u>
History. Sexual history, previous birth control method, level of motivation.

<u>Objective</u>
Physical Examination. Pelvic exam. Note vaginal muscle tone and depth of notch behind symphysis pubis, breast exam as indicated.

Lab. Normal Pap smear within previous 6 months, test for sexually transmitted diseases if indicated.

<u>Assessment</u>. Determine suitability of method for individual's need. Determine if contraindications exist. Assess patient's dexterity. Contraindications would include uterine prolapse, cystocele, rectocele, vaginal fistula, or septa, reluctance of patient to touch genitals or lack of motivation to use consistently. **Complications** include allergic reaction to spermicide, UTI, and pregnancy.

PLAN/MANAGEMENT PROTOCOL
General Measures. Teach patient how to insert and remove diaphragm. Recheck patient and assess patient's skill and comfort at inserting and removing. Complete instructions on use, spermicide use, length of time spermicide is active, length of time following intercourse diaphragm must be used, how to add additional spermicide if necessary. Instruct patient on proper care of diaphragm. Emphasize and re-emphasize **safe sex practices** and educate about the use of condoms.

Specific Measures. Diaphragm of choice and appropriate size
_____*(MIS)
                                         or
_____*(MIS).

Physician Consultation. Consider if adverse reaction, complications, or anatomic abnormalities.

Referral.

Follow-up Plan. Usually in _____ weeks to check for patient's ability to insert and use appropriately. Subsequently, recheck in _____ months, sooner if problems occur.

			Initials	Date
* unless allergic, contraindicated,		Physician		
or pregnant/lactating		ARNP		

Vaginal Spermicides and Contraceptive Sponges

EVALUATION/DIAGNOSTIC PROTOCOL
Subjective
History. Sexual history, gynecologic history, motivation and needs.

Objective
Physical Examination. As indicated.

Lab. As indicated.

Assess appropriateness for individual. Possible contraindications include allergy to spermicide, discomfort in touching genitals, lack of motivation for consistent use. In the case of the vaginal sponge, history of Toxic Shock Syndrome would be contraindication for use as well as some anatomic abnormalities. **Complications.** Method failure and unwanted pregnancy, hypersensitivity to spermicide or sponge.

PLAN/MANAGEMENT PROTOCOL
General Measures. Advise patient to read instructions on package. Plan well to insert proper mixing of spermicide with foam. Emphasize and re-emphasize **safe sex practices** and educate about the use of condoms.
　　Foam: instruct patient on proper insertion, reinsertion, and care of applicator.
　　Suppositories: have patient insert high inside vagina and wait for the correct amount of time as directed on package instructions.
　　Vaginal sponges: advise patient to moisten sponge and insert to cover the cervix. Check placement before and after intercourse and leave in for _____ hours (to avoid Toxic Shock Syndrome). Advise of over-the-counter availability and need for use with each intercourse. Strongly recommend routine use of condoms to prevent STD transmission.

Physician Consultation. If there is any question of Toxic Shock Syndrome.

Referral.

Follow-up Plan. Consider individual or couple follow-up visit in _____ weeks if birth control method has been difficult issue.

	Initials	Date
* unless allergic, contraindicated, or pregnant/lactating	Physician ARNP	

Fertility Awareness Method

EVALUATION/DIAGNOSTIC PROTOCOL
<u>Subjective</u>
History. Sexual and gynecological history, level of motivation and degree of effectiveness needed.

<u>Objective</u>
Physical Examination. As indicated.

Lab. As indicated.

Assess suitability and determine if contraindications exist. Possible contraindications include irregular intervals between menses, history of anovulatory cycles, breast feeding, lack of motivation and unstable lifestyle. **Complications**. Method failure and unwanted pregnancy.

PLAN/MANAGEMENT PROTOCOL
General Measures. The instructions for using this method should be thorough and optimally given to the couple rather than just an individual. The practitioner should be educated in all three areas (BBT, calendar method, and the mucus changes) before attempting counseling. Patient handout materials should be provided to assist proper record-keeping and for reminder of instructions. Records should be kept for at least 6 consecutive menstrual cycles before a couple attempts to rely on this method alone. This method may be used to assist in planning as well as preventing conception. It does not suffice for preventing STD transmission. Emphasize and re-emphasize **safe sex practices** and educate about the use of condoms.

Physician Consultation. Usually not necessary unless having difficulty interpreting patient's chart.

Referral. In cases of infertility pending physician consult if no success with fertility awareness counseling alone.

Follow-up Plan. Follow-up visit in _____ months or as indicated to assist patient in interpreting charted results and evaluating continued motivation.

	Initials	Date
Physician		
ARNP		

* unless allergic, contraindicated,
or pregnant/lactating

Menopause

EVALUATION/DIAGNOSTIC PROTOCOL
Subjective
History. Complete gynecologic and obstetrical history (course of menstrual change, usually oligomenorrhea and increased or irregular interval between menses). Any symptoms of vasomotor instability (hot flashes and sweats)? Genitourinary symptoms (dyspareunia, vulval dryness and/or pruritis, dysuria)? Any general symptoms (depression, fatigue, irritability)? Family history.

Objective
Physical Examination. General appearance, vital signs, thyroid, chest, breasts, cardiovascular, abdomen, pelvic (kraurosis vulvae, vaginal mucosal changes, cervical atrophy), rectal.

Lab. Pap smear (increased superficial cells) and FSH (increased).

Assess severity of symptomatology. **Differential Diagnosis.** Pregnancy, other endocrine causes (hypothyroidism), psychologic causes, other physiologic causes (marked exercise increase, drastically decreased nutritional state). **Complications.** Worsening of symptoms discussed above, include the significant long term problem of osteoporosis (see Osteoporosis) and probable increased risk for atherosclerotic vascular disease.

PLAN/MANAGEMENT PROTOCOL
General Measures. Be sensitive to the patient's concerns. Explain menopause. Assess the patient's risk for osteoporosis (see Osteoporosis). Recommend estrogen replacement therapy to those who are symptomatic or have physical signs, or are at risk for complications and who do not have contraindications:

Absolute contraindications are those with known or suspected breast cancer, estrogen-dependent neoplasms, pregnancy, undiagnosed vaginal bleeding, or history of thrombophlebitis or thromboembolism associated with estrogen use.

Relative contraindications are widely debated and the authors encourage the nurse practitioner and physician consultant or supervisor to establish some choices for their patients amongst these (or individualize for each patient). These include: other history of or active vascular thrombosis, strong family history of breast cancer, fibrocystic breast disease, hypertension, coronary artery disease, cerebral vascular disease, migraine and the other vascular headaches, certain hepatic disorders, known estrogen intolerance, strong family history of endometrial carcinoma.

Patients must be informed about possible increased risk of endometrial carcinoma on replacement.

Specific Measures
Estrogen replacement therapy _____*(MIS)

or

alternative estrogen therapy _____*(MIS).

Consider progestin therapy _____*(MIS).

Physician Consultation. Consider for new patients. Any patient developing a complication of therapy.

Follow-up Plan. Recheck in _____ months to include BP, weight, lipid panel and review of tolerance of therapy. Subsequently, recheck every _____ months. Immediate if unexpected bleeding (emphasize to patient) and as needed for other concerns.

		Initials	Date
* unless allergic, contraindicated,	Physician		
or pregnant/lactating	ARNP		

CHAPTER 10
ORTHOPEDICS

Lumbosacral Strain

EVALUATION/DIAGNOSTIC PROTOCOL
Subjective
History. Description of pain: onset, frequency, duration, radiation, precipitating factors, location, and chronicity. Any systemic symptoms or other indications of arthritis. History of trauma or overuse. Family history.

Objective
Physical Examination. General appearance, complete back exam, peripheral pulses, appropriate neuro exam.

Lab. Usually none. May need lumbosacral spine x-rays and/or EMGs.

Assess severity and signs of radiculopathy. **Differential Diagnosis.** If no radiculopathy, consider GYN infection, genitourinary infection, vascular disorders, or depression. **Complications.** Disk herniation. Chronic back pain affecting family, job, social situation.

PLAN/MANAGEMENT PROTOCOL
General Measures. For acute strain, bed rest for at least 2-3 days. Ice massage for localized tenderness. For chronic low back pain, limit activity, especially lifting. Application of warm, moist heat for 20 minutes intermittently. Patient education on proper stretching, strengthening exercises, and prevention of back strain. Provide or recommend reinforcing educational material (such as Back Care by Consumer Reports).

Specific Measures. None. Non-steroidal anti-inflammatory drug of choice. OTC
_____*(MIS)

or

_____*(MIS).

Consider muscle relaxant _____*(MIS)

or

_____*(MIS).

Consider narcotic analgesic for severe pain _____*(MIS).

Physician Consultation. Consider whenever there is a history of injury and potential litigation. Consider if in severe pain or if signs of radiculopathy. Consider if patient not improving significantly within 1-2 weeks.

Referral.
May need EMGs and neurology consult.
Orthopedic referral for persistent or severe chronic back pain.
Consider therapeutic massage or physical therapy when appropriate.

Immediate Transfer.

Follow-up Plan. Follow up by phone in _____ days and in _____ weeks in office as indicated.

	Initials	Date
* unless allergic, contraindicated, or pregnant/lactating	Physician ARNP	

Cervical Neck Sprain

EVALUATION/DIAGNOSTIC PROTOCOL
Subjective
History. Specific injury or secondary to overuse or prolonged unconscious muscle contraction, accompanying symptoms.

Objective
Physical Examination. General appearance, musculoskeletal exam of neck, arms, shoulders, and upper back; peripheral pulses, appropriate neuro exam.

Lab. X-ray with history of injury, especially if there is possibility of litigation. Be sure radiologic written report is obtained.

Assess whether simple cervical strain, acute or recurrent. **Differential Diagnosis.** Underlying pathology, including congenital malformation and neoplasm. **Complications.** Complete ligamentous tear, disk rupture, dislocation, spinal cord injury, fracture, lymphadenopathy, meningitis, or angina.

PLAN/MANAGEMENT PROTOCOL
General Measures. Rest, application of soft cervical collar when appropriate. Ice packs for 20 minutes intermittently during first 24 hours, then warm, moist heat for 20 minutes intermittently. Gentle massage. Patient education re: stretching and relaxation exercises for neck and shoulders, course of healing, and prevention.

Specific Measures. Non-steroidal anti-inflammatory drug of choice

_____*(MIS)

or

_____*(MIS).

Consider muscle relaxant _____*(MIS)

or

_____*(MIS).

Consider narcotic analgesic for severe pain _____*(MIS).

Physician Consultation. Consider within 24 hours with history of injury or auto accident and potential litigation. Consider if patient shows no improvement within 48 hours. Consider if any signs of nerve impingement.

Referral.
May need EMGs and neurology consult.
Orthopedic referral for persistent or severe chronic neck pain.
Consider therapeutic massage or physical therapy when appropriate.

Immediate Transfer. If disk rupture, dislocation, or spinal cord injury are suspected. Stabilize neck and back to prevent movement during transfer.

Follow-up Plan. In _____ hours if no improvement, otherwise in _____ week(s) when indicated.

	Initials	Date
* unless allergic, contraindicated,	Physician	
or pregnant/lactating	ARNP	

Ankle Sprain

EVALUATION/DIAGNOSTIC PROTOCOL

Subjective

History. Description of injury and symptoms (acute, chronic, or recurrent). Frequency of sports activity/exercise program.

Objective

Physical Examination. Complete joint exam, pulses, and appropriate neuro exam.

Lab. Consider x-ray.

Assessment. Ankle sprains may be classified into three grades: grade I, stretching of involved ligaments; grade II, partial tearing of involved ligaments with slight joint instability; grade III, severe ligament tearing with loss of stability. Differential Diagnosis is essentially amongst the types of sprains, but be careful to evaluate for predisposing conditions. Complications. Instability.

PLAN/MANAGEMENT PROTOCOL

General Measures. Ice pack ankle for 20 minutes off and on for 48 hours.

Elastic bandage to control swelling and provide stability. Elevate ankle. Crutches for at least 2-3 days, depending on severity.

Patient education re: type of injury and healing time, strengthening exercises, and prevention.

Specific Measures. Analgesic or non-steroidal anti-inflammatory drug of choice.
_____*(MIS)
                                    or
_____*(MIS).

Physician Consultation. Consider for grade II or grade III sprains or when in doubt about severity or need for x-ray. When an eversion injury due to increased risk for bony damage and tearing of deltoid and inferior tibiofibular ligaments If not significantly improved in 24 hours.

Referral.
Orthopedic referral for persistent or severe pain, joint instability or fracture. Consider physical therapy and rehabilitation program.

Immediate Transfer. If the joint is unstable and fracture is suspected.

Follow-up Plan. Follow up in _____ hour(s) or as indicated, or if not significantly improved after initial follow-up visit. Additional follow-up every _____ week(s) as indicated.

	Initials	Date
* unless allergic, contraindicated, or pregnant/lactating	Physician ARNP	

Knee Sprain

EVALUATION/DIAGNOSTIC PROTOCOL
<u>Subjective</u>
History. Description of injury: when, how, was there immediate swelling or instability? Previous history of knee problems? Frequency of sports activity, exercise program.

<u>Objective</u>
Physical Examination. Complete joint exam. Check peripheral pulses and appropriate neuro exam.

Lab. Consider x-ray.

<u>Assess</u> severity: mild or minor (first and second degree) ligamentous injury; whether medial or lateral collateral or cruciate ligament is sprained. **Differential Diagnosis** among the various ligamentous injuries as well as cartilage or bony injury. **Complications.** Complete ligamentous tear or third-degree sprain, meniscal tear, fracture, or other joint capsule damage.

<u>PLAN</u>/**MANAGEMENT PROTOCOL**
General Measures. Elevation of knee with application of ice for 20 minutes intermittent for 24-48 hours. Compression bandages and use of crutches to avoid weight-bearing. Patient education re: isometric quadriceps and hamstrings exercises, course of healing, and prevention. Provide/prescribe immobilizer if concerned about internal derangement.

Specific Measures. Analgesic or non-steroidal anti-inflammatory drug of choice
_____*(MIS)
or
_____*(MIS).

Physician Consultation. Consider if there is presence of significant hemorrhage and joint effusion or any question of joint instability or internal derangement.

Referral.
Orthopedic referral for persistent or severe pain, joint instability or fracture. Consider physical therapy and rehabilitation program.

Immediate Transfer. Immediately if fracture or complete ligamentous tear is suspected, or if septic joint is suspected, to orthopedic surgeon.

Follow-up Plan. Usually in _____ weeks. Often not necessary with mild knee sprain.

	Initials	Date
* unless allergic, contraindicated, or pregnant/lactating	Physician ARNP	

Dislocations

EVALUATION/DIAGNOSTIC PROTOCOL
Subjective
History. History of injury and accompanying symptoms. Previous history of similar dislocations.

Objective
Physical Examination. Observe injured part. Do not attempt to reduce dislocation before x-rays are taken.

Lab. X-rays should always be taken.

Assess extent of dislocation. **Differential Diagnosis**. Ligament, cartilage, or bony injury. **Complications**. Neurologic or vascular injury, permanent impairment, potential for impending shock.

PLAN/MANAGEMENT PROTOCOL
General Measures. Usually these patients will present at hospital. If they are in severe pain and have obvious dislocation, immediate ambulance transfer is indicated. If patient is in mild to moderate pain and dislocation is suspected, send for x-ray and consult with physician. Dislocations that may be handled by the nurse practitioner with physician consultation include:

_____

_____

_____.

After reduction and immobilization, splint should be used for _____ weeks as indicated. Patient education about prevention of repeat dislocations, follow-up care, and isometric exercises.

Specific Measures.
Drug of choice for pain _____*(MIS)
                                          or
_____*(MIS).

Physician Consultation. Consider whenever dislocation is obvious or suspected and management not previously determined by protocol or responding to treatment.

Referral.

Immediate Transfer. As indicated by severity of dislocation and pain.

Follow-up Plan. Depending on type of dislocation, may be from _____ days to _____ weeks.

	Initials	Date

* unless allergic, contraindicated,   Physician
or pregnant/lactating   ARNP

Fractures

EVALUATION/DIAGNOSTIC PROTOCOL
<u>Subjective</u>
History. History of injury and description of symptoms.

<u>Objective</u>
Physical Examination. Careful exam of injured extremity or area, vital signs, assess for impending shock.

Lab. Always x-ray with suspicion of fracture.

<u>Assess</u> type of fracture(s) and location. **Differential Diagnosis.** Soft tissue injury, periosteal contusion, bony contusion. **Complications.** Temporary or permanent functional impairment, neurologic or vascular injury, potential for impending shock.

PLAN/MANAGEMENT PROTOCOL
General Measures. If injury is severe, control of pain and shock are indicated until patient can be transferred to hospital. Always splint the injured part during transfer process. Check circulation and vital signs as indicated. If injury is not severe, have patient sent for x-rays with wet reading. Alert supervising physician. Fractures of the following bones may be handled by the nurse practitioner with physician consultation:

_____
_____
_____.

Patient education re: course of healing, care of cast or other immobilization device, and follow-up plan.

Specific Measures. Drug of choice for severe pain or shock during immediate transfer with severe fracture _____*(MIS).

Drug of choice for pain relief with simple fractures that are managed in primary care office _____*(MIS)
                                    or
_____*(MIS).

Physician Consultation. Whenever a fracture is suspected and not covered by protocols.

Referral. Pending physician consultation for follow-up with orthopedic surgeon. Casting is to be done _____.

Immediate Transfer. For all severe fractures, call ambulance immediately while stabilizing patient, splinting fracture and assessing for shock.

Follow-up Plan. As indicated by treatment. May include _____.

	Initials	Date
* unless allergic, contraindicated, or pregnant/lactating	Physician ARNP	

Degenerative Joint Disease

EVALUATION/DIAGNOSTIC PROTOCOL

Subjective

History. Description of symptoms with attention to location of pain and length of early morning stiffness, if present. Systemic symptoms, if any. Review concurrent medical conditions, current medications, and drug allergies.

Objective

Physical Examination. Thorough musculoskeletal exam, including all joints, weight, and height.

Lab. Consider x-rays, CBC, sedimentation rate, RA latex, ANA, uric acid as indicated.

Assess degree of functional impairment of involved joints. **Differential Diagnosis.** Inflammatory arthritis, strains and sprains, tendonitis or bursitis. **Complications.** Worsening joint function, chronic pain, and those complications that relate to significant immobility.

PLAN/MANAGEMENT PROTOCOL

General Measures. Rest involved joints, physical therapy, including corrective exercises, elimination of trauma, including weight loss or occupational adjustment. Occasionally back or neck supports are helpful. Patient education about disease course and outcome including weight loss program when appropriate. Provide or recommend reinforcing educational materials (such as Exercise for Arthritis by Consumer Reports). Some patients will need appliances to assist with ambulation or activities of daily living.

Specific Measures. Analgesic or non-steroidal anti-inflammatory agents of choice
_____*(MIS)
or
_____*(MIS)
or
_____*(MIS).

Consider Rx _____*(MIS)
to protect upper GI tract from NSAID.

Physician Consultation. Consider if unable to rule out septic or inflammatory arthritis or if there is neurological involvement or significant disability.

Referral. Consider for physical therapy, orthopedic, or rheumatologic consultation where appropriate.

Immediate Transfer. None.

Follow-up Plan. Every _____ months or more frequently if assisting patient with lifestyle modification.

	Initials	Date
* unless allergic, contraindicated, or pregnant/lactating	Physician ARNP	

CHAPTER 11
DERMATOLOGY

Acne

EVALUATION/DIAGNOSTIC PROTOCOL
Subjective
History. Patient's description, course of symptoms, patient's perceptions about cause, treatment and, most significantly, self-image. Family history. Previous medications used.

Objective
Physical Examination. Thorough examination of the skin, lesion types (non-inflammatory blackheads, whiteheads) and inflammatory red papules, pustules, cysts and scars.

Lab. None.

Assess severity and type: non-inflammatory, inflammatory. **Differential Diagnosis.** Furunculosis, rosacea. **Complications.** Secondary infection, self-image, and emotional disturbance.

PLAN/MANAGEMENT PROTOCOL
General Measures. Reassurance that acne can be managed. Wash involved areas with mild soap and water (abrasive soaps and astringents not necessary, can be irritating). Avoid oil-based cosmetics. Recommend wearing hair up off the face. Eat a balanced diet and drink plenty of water. It is usually not necessary to avoid any foods. Discourage "picking of pimples." See Acne Care instruction sheet.

Specific Measures.

Benzoyl peroxide OTC or Rx _____*(MIS)
                                          and/or
consider topical tretinoin Rx _____*(MIS)
                                          and/or

topical antibiotic Rx _____*(MIS).

For inflammatory lesions antibiotic therapy, oral Rx _____

_____*(MIS).

CAUTION: The authors recommend limited use of Accutane to established protocols.

Physician Consultation. Consider for severe, inflammatory acne or complications. Or for therapeutic failure or intolerance of treatment.

Referral.

Follow-up Plan. _____ weeks initially and then intervally every _____ weeks/ months, or as needed.

                                                            Initials   Date

* unless allergic, containdicated   Physician
or pregnant/lactating   ARNP

Rosacea

EVALUATION/DIAGNOSTIC PROTOCOL

Subjective

History. Patient's description, course of symptoms (blushing easily), patient's perceptions about cause, treatment and, most significantly, self-image. Family history.

Objective

Physical Examination. Thorough examination of the skin, lesion types (erythema middle third of face, inflammatory red papules, pustules, cysts and rhinophyma).

Lab. None.

Assess severity of erythema (recurrent or persistent with/without telangiectasia) and severity of rhinophyma. **Differential Diagnosis.** Cellulitis, furunculosis, acne vulgaris. **Complications.** Secondary infection, self-image and emotional disturbance.

PLAN/MANAGEMENT PROTOCOL

General Measures. Explain that the cause is unknown, that this is more common in fair skinned individuals and unrelated to chronic alcohol use (W. C. Fields gave it a bad name). Explain further that this disease has periods of activity and inactivity.

Recommend moisturizers, mild soaps/cleansers, and sunscreens while avoiding typical acne medicines which might exacerbate dryness. See Dry Skin Information Sheet.

The patient should avoid those things which seem to aggravate his/her condition. These things include drinking hot liquids which contribute to facial flushing and may include spicy foods, alcohol, stress, sunlight and temperature extremes.

Therapy is directed at controlling symptoms and slowing or even halting progression. The patient should be told cure is unlikely.

Specific Measures.

Oral antibiotic Rx _____ *(MIS)

                                       or

alternative oral antibiotic Rx _____ *(MIS)

                                    and/or

topical antibiotic Rx _____ *(MIS).

_____ *(MIS).

Physician Consultation. Consider for severe, rosacea or complications. Or for therapeutic failure or intolerance of treatment.

Referral. To dermatologist for severe or refractory disease.

Follow-up Plan. _____ weeks initially and then intervally every _____ weeks or as needed.

	Initials	Date
* unless allergic, containdicated or pregnant/lactating	Physician ARNP	

Pruritis

EVALUATION/DIAGNOSTIC PROTOCOL

<u>Subjective</u>

History. Symptoms, course (aggravating and alleviating circumstances). Ask patient about environmental, occupational, hobby or habit risks. Family history, similar symptoms, and/or allergic diseases. Be attentive to psycho-emotional etiology. Any constitutional symptoms (amendmentitis, preambleopia, conventional wisdom!)?

<u>Objective</u>

Physical Examination. Thorough skin examination. (If no historical or dermatologic cause, then complete physical exam should be done)

Lab. Consider CBC, chemistry profile, thyroid survey, U/A, stool for O&P.

<u>Assessment</u> is focused on etiology as well as severity. **Differential Diagnosis** beyond dermatologic causes includes drug allergy, occult infection, parasites, renal failure, biliary obstruction (OCPs or pregnancy), occult malignancy, anemia and commonly psychoneurologic causes.

PLAN/MANAGEMENT PROTOCOL

General Measures. Avoid detergents, soaps, and extended bathing, which dry the skin. Avoid irritating bedding and clothing. For specifically itchy area, consider ice water compress or gentle ice massage. Soothing tepid to cool baths with the addition of colloidal oatmeal.

Consider antipruritic lotions or emulsions _____
_____ or _____.

Specific Measures.

Consider oral antihistamine OTC or Rx _____*(MIS)
                                    or
alternative antihistamine (even H-2) Rx _____*(MIS).

Limited course of topical corticosteroids OTC or Rx _____*(MIS)
                                    or
alternative topical corticosteroid Rx _____*(MIS).

Physician Consultation. Consider for severe disease, suspected underlying pathology, treatment failure, or suspected psycho-social etiology.

Referral.

Follow-up Plan. Every _____ week(s), sooner if needed.

Initials   Date

* unless allergic, containdicated   Physician
or pregnant/lactating   ARNP

Acute Urticaria

EVALUATION/DIAGNOSTIC PROTOCOL
<u>Subjective</u>
History. Symptoms, course (aggravating and alleviating circumstances). Ask about foods, environmental changes, occupation, hobby and habit exposures. Review use of all medications.   Family history of similar problem or allergic disorders.
Any other constitutional symptoms (fever, arthralgias)?

<u>Objective</u>
Physical Examination. General, vital signs, and skin. Consider close examination of all mucosal surfaces for possible clue as to etiology including streptococcal pharyngitis and candidal vulvovaginitis.

Lab. Not necessary initially except for one of the afore-mentioned causes.
Consider _____ for persistent symptomatology.

<u>Assess</u> severity, and if generalized reaction or respiratory distress (see <u>Anaphylaxis</u>). **Differential Diagnosis** is directed at etiology though this is not found in over 50% of patients. If arthralgias or arthritis, consider other systemic illness. **Complications**. Serum sickness and anaphylaxis.

PLAN/MANAGEMENT PROTOCOL
General Measures. Remember that careful history often reveals etiology and to consequently remind the patient to keep looking for likely causes.
    Ice water compressing or gentle ice massage or cool baths. Specifically, avoid hot baths and showers.

Specific Measures.
Consider antihistamine, oral OTC or Rx _____*(MIS)

or

alternative or additional antihistamine (even H-2) _____*(MIS).

With chronicity, consider low dose antidepressant _____*(MIS).

Physician Consultation. Consider for severe urticaria, suspected neoplasm or other underlying pathology, treatment failure or complications.

Referral.

Immediate Transfer. If signs or symptoms of potential respiratory distress.

Follow-up Plan. Recheck in _____ days, sooner if worse. Caution patient or parent about signs that warrant immediate reattention.

	Initials	Date
* unless allergic, containdicated	Physician	
or pregnant/lactating	ARNP	

Contact Dermatitis

EVALUATION/DIAGNOSTIC PROTOCOL
<u>Subjective</u>
History. Symptoms, course (initial appearance, ascertain possible exposure to irritant or allergen as well as aggravating and alleviating factors).

<u>Objective</u>
Physical Examination. Thorough skin examination note location and distribution of (in order of severity from minimum to maximum) erythema, vesicles, blisters, erosions, ulcers. Patches and streaks are the sine qua non.

Lab. Usually not necessary, though consideration should be given to herpes culture.

Assess severity and possible etiology. **Differential Diagnosis.** Atopic, seborrheic, and other vesicular/bullous dermatoses, dermatophyte infections and scabies. **Complications.** Excoriations and secondary infections.

PLAN/MANAGEMENT PROTOCOL
General Measures. Remove the irritant. In the future avoid the contact allergen. Emphasize to the patient that even with treatment it may be several weeks before resolution occurs. Use only mild soaps when washing.
    Cold compressing _____.
    Soothing creams and lotions _____
_____.

Specific Measures.
Consider oral antihistamine OTC and Rx _____*(MIS).

Consider corticosteroid, topical OTC or Rx _____*(MIS)

Be certain to limit use and potency on young children and on any face or other area likely to be damaged permanently.
or

Short course oral Rx CHILD _____

Or ADULT _____*(MIS).

Physician Consultation. Consider for severe cases, therapeutic complications, therapeutic failure or diagnostic doubt.

Referral.

Immediate Transfer. May be necessary for caustic contactants.

Follow-up Plan. _____ days if no improvement, sooner if worse.

<table>
<tr><td></td><td>Initials</td><td>Date</td></tr>
<tr><td>* unless allergic, containdicated
or pregnant/lactating</td><td>Physician
ARNP</td><td></td></tr>
</table>

Atopic Dermatitis

EVALUATION/DIAGNOSTIC PROTOCOL
Subjective
History. Symptoms, course (aggravating and alleviating factors), long-term history (infant, child, adolescent, adult phases). Family history, allergic disorders, previous attempts at treatment and response.

Objective
Physical Examination. Complete skin exam. Consider ENT and respiratory exam.

Lab. Necessary only if secondary infection suspected persistent/refractory.

Assess severity. **Differential Diagnosis.** Contact or seborrheic dermatitis, psoriasis **Complications** are secondary infections.

PLAN/MANAGEMENT PROTOCOL
General Measures. Explain to parent or patient this is hypersensitive skin that dries out easily, causing itching, which is controllable but not curable. Avoid detergents, soaps, and extended bathing which dry the skin. Avoid irritating bedding and clothing. See Dry Skin Information Sheet. Employ OTC topical moisterizers and emollients after bathing that seal in moisture before toweling dry. Consider the addition of a multivitamin mineral supplement to the diet.

Specific Measures.
Consider intermittent use of topical corticosteroids OTC or Rx

_____ and/or _____ *(MIS).

Consider oral antihistamine OTC or Rx _____ *(MIS).

Consider oral antibiotic Rx _____ *(MIS)
                                    and/or
consider topical antibiotic Rx _____ *(MIS).

Physician Consultation. Consider for severe disease or treatment failure.

Referral. To dermatologist if no improvement in _____ weeks.

Immediate Transfer. Usually not necessary.

Follow-up Plan. Every _____ week(s) during active phase and every _____ weeks, months subsequently, or as needed.

Initials   Dat

* unless allergic, contraindicated   Physician
or pregnant/lactating   ARNP

Diaper Dermatitis

EVALUATION/DIAGNOSTIC PROTOCOL
Subjective
History. Symptoms, course, predisposing factors (diaper type, occlusive pants, cleansing practices, changing frequency, recent antibiotic usage), underlying conditions.

Objective
Physical Examination. Complete physical. Specific location (lower trunk and band-like, contact surfaces, creases, perianal). Satellite lesions?

Lab. Consider KOH prep.

Assess severity. **Differential Diagnosis.** After excluding atopy, the key to distinguishing among the common causes is the pattern and location (contact surfaces due to ammonia or contactants, creases due to moisture maceration, perianal from acid stools, candida anywhere but typically with satellite lesions). **Complications.** Excoriations and secondary infection.

PLAN/MANAGEMENT PROTOCOL
General Measures. Allow air circulation whenever possible even by not diapering. When diapering, change frequently, washing diaper area with warm water. If needed, use only mild soap. Stop (temporarily or permanently) occlusive pants or disposable diapers. Switch to cloth diapers be sure to wash in mild detergent and to rinse thoroughly. If ammonia is in diapers then add vinegar to rinse water. Discontinue use of ointments, cleansers and lotions, especially disposable wipes. If perianal, try dabbing area with dilute baking soda solution.

Specific Measures.
May recommend specific OTC preparation _____.

If candida, recommend topical antifungal Otc/Rx _____.

And if recent antibiotic use consider oral mycostatin _____*(MIS).

Physician Consultation. Consider if severe, recurring or suspected neglect,

Referral.

Immediate Transfer.

Follow-up Plan. Recheck if not improved in _____ days.

	Initials	Date
* unless allergic, containdicated	Physician	
or pregnant/lactating	ARNP	

Seborrheic Dermatitis

EVALUATION/DIAGNOSTIC PROTOCOL
Subjective
History. Symptoms, course (aggravating and alleviating factors, long-term history) Family history.

Objective
Physical Examination. Complete skin exam with attention to scalp, other hairy or creased areas.

Lab. None necessary.

Assess severity. **Differential Diagnosis.** Atopic and contact dermatitis, psoriasis, **Complications.** Excoriations.

PLAN/MANAGEMENT PROTOCOL
General Measures. Reassure patient this is not contagious.

Discuss that therapeutic measures are directed at controlling scaling/flaking. In infants with cradle cap, consider applying olive oil 15 minutes before mild shampooing and gentle brushing 3 times a week.

Specific Measures. For adults and children over 2 years.
Selenium sulfide shampoo to scalp _____*(MIS).
Zinc pyrithione shampoo _____*(MIS).

Consider topical corticosteroid, OTC or Rx _____*(MIS).
Sprays most effective in hairy areas.

If evidence of secondary infection, treat with oral antibiotic Rx _____
_____*(MIS). (Be aware of candidiasis as a possible infection before or after antibiotic usage. Also be aware that recent research shows occult dermatophyte infections common. Consider topical antifungal.)

Physician Consultation. Consider for severe disease, treatment failure, refractory infection.

Referral. To dermatologist if no improvement in _____ weeks.

Immediate Transfer. Usually not necessary.

Follow-up Plan. Every _____ weeks during active phase and every _____ weeks/months subsequently. Sooner if worse.

```
                                                Initials      Date
* unless allergic, containdicated       Physician
  or pregnant/lactating                 ARNP
```

Psoriasis

EVALUATION/DIAGNOSTIC PROTOCOL
Subjective
History. Patient's description of lesion or rash. Course of symptoms (initial appearance, long term variation, aggravating and alleviating circumstances. Associated local (itching) and generalized (constitutional and/cr of arthritis) symptoms. Family history.

Objective
Physical Examination. General appearance, vital signs, joints. Because of extraordinary variability thorough skin exam (classically--circumscribed plaque with fine silvery scale on erythematous base, guttate--small scattered tear-drops, exfoliative--generalized).

Lab. CBC, chemistry panel, sed rate, RPR. Consider biopsy and or x-ray hands or other joints.

Assess type, extent, and severity. This is a chronic relapsing and variable disorder, carefully work through the **Differential Diagnosis**, including atopic, contact and seborrheic dermatitis, drug eruption, secondary syphilis, pityriasis rosea, tinea corporis and versicolor. **Complications.** Significant arthritic destruction.

PLAN/MANAGEMENT PROTOCOL
General Measures. Explain to patient that cause is unknown, appear to autoimmune mediated and by considerable variability and relapses.

Encourage sunlight in moderate amounts. Caution about skin injury which can become new site of psoriasis.

Review skin care measures, including good hygiene but avoiding drying cleansers (see <u>Dry Skin</u> information sheet).

Provide reinforcing educational materials.

Specific Measures.
Consider topical corticosteroid _____*(MIS).

Consider coal tar topicals _____*(MIS).

Consider topical anthration _____*(MIS).

Physician Consultation. Consider for diagnostic uncertainty, severe or refractory cases.

Referral. Consider dermatologist _____.

Immediate Transfer.

Follow-up Plan. Initially every _____ weeks/months and subsequently every _____ months or as needed.

	Initials	Date
Physician		
ARNP		

* unless allergic, containdicated
or pregnant/lactating

Pityriasis rosea

EVALUATION/DIAGNOSTIC PROTOCOL
<u>Subjective</u>
History. General and skin history, onset and course of symptoms with particular attention to the "herald patch."

<u>Objective</u>
Physical Examination. General appearance, vital signs, lymphoreticular exam, microsal surface, and complete skin exam.

Lab. CBC and consider RPR (or VDRL).

<u>Assessment</u> is directed at **Differential Diagnosis**, which includes drug eruption, secondary syphilis, tinea corporis, tinea versicolor, seborrhea, psoriasis. **Complications.** None.

PLAN/MANAGEMENT PROTOCOL
General Measures. Be sure to explain the benign nature of this condition and that it may last 3-12 weeks to patient and/or parents. Cold water compressing or gentle ice massage is soothing. When bathing add baking soda or colloidal oatmeal.

Specific Measures. No specific therapy.
Consider antipruritic OTC or Rx _____*(MIS).

Physician Consultation. Consider depending upon severity or uncertainty of diagnosis.

Referral.

Immediate Transfer. Usually not necessary.

Follow-up Plan. Recheck in _____ weeks.

Initials   Date

* unless allergic, containdicated   Physician
or pregnant/lactating   ARNP

Impetigo

EVALUATION/DIAGNOSTIC PROTOCOL
<u>Subjective</u>
History. Symptoms and course (pustules vs. blisters/bullae).

<u>Objective</u>
Physical Examination. Describe lesions, stage and location. (Pustules become honey-colored crusts on erythematous base while vesicles and bullae go from flat, flaccid and clear to tense and cloudy, then thin-crusted or are superficial ulcerations on an erythematous base (burn-like).

Lab. Cultures rarely necessary except when differential diagnosis confusing.

<u>Assessment</u> distinguishes nonbullous streptococcal vs. bullous staphylococcal impetigo. **Differential Diagnosis**. Insect bites and herpes simplex. **Complications**. Acute glomerulonephritis.

PLAN/MANAGEMENT PROTOCOL
General Measures. Advise patient or parents that over-the-counter topical therapy is ineffective.
Wash affected areas thoroughly with soap and water, gently scrubbing crusts 4 times a day. Keep children's fingernails cut short. Clothing, towels, washcloths and bedding should be washed daily. Encourage meticulous family hygiene.

Specific Measures Oral antibiotic Rx _____*(MIS)
                                         or

alternative antibiotic Rx _____*(MIS).

Consider IM injection benzathine penicillin.

Consider recommending OTC or prescription antibacterial cleanser _____.

Physician Consultation. Consider for very severe, frequent recurrences, suspected neglect, acute glomerulonephritis.

Referral.

Immediate Transfer.

Follow-up Plan. _____ days if not improved, sooner if worse or if sequalae.

	Initials	Date

* unless allergic, containdicated   Physician
or pregnant/lactating   ARNP

Furuncles and Carbuncles

EVALUATION/DIAGNOSTIC PROTOCOL
<u>Subjective</u>
History. History of contributing factors, course and location.

<u>Objective</u>
Physical Examination. Complete skin exam. Lesion size and location, presence or absence of lymphangitis or lymphadenopathy.

Lab. Not necessary, usually staphylococcal.

<u>Assess</u> severity. **Differential Diagnosis.** Insect bites, foreign body site. **Complications.** Bacteremia.

PLAN/MANAGEMENT PROTOCOL
General Measures. Hot compressing 10-20 minutes 4 times a day. Bathe head to toe twice daily.

Keep fingernails short.

Clothing, towels, washcloth and bedding should be washed daily.

Meticulous family hygiene.

Specific Measures. Large fluctuant carbuncles should be incised and drained.

Consider oral antibiotic Rx _____ *(MIS)
                                                        or
alternative antibiotic Rx _____ *(MIS).

Physician Consultation. Consider for unusual or severe lesions, treatment failure, referral to surgeon.

Referral.

Immediate Transfer.

Follow-up Plan. Recheck in _____ days if not improved, sooner if worse. Recheck I. and D.'s hours, if packing placed or as indicated.

Initials   Date

* unless allergic, containdicated   Physician
or pregnant/lactating   ARNP

Cellulitis/Folliculitis

EVALUATION/DIAGNOSTIC PROTOCOL
<u>Subjective</u>
History. Symptoms and course. Note predisposing situations or underlying conditions.

<u>Objective</u>
Physical Examination. General appearance, vital signs, area involved (size and location), lymphangitis or lymph adenopathy.

Lab. Consider culture and sensitivity.

<u>Assess</u> severity. **Differential Diagnosis.** Impetigo. **Complications.** Bacteremia.

<u>PLAN/MANAGEMENT PROTOCOL</u>
General Measures. Wash affected area with soap and water 4 times a day.

Avoid or modify predisposing circumstances.

Meticulous family hygiene.

Clothing, towels, washcloth, bedding should be washed daily.

Specific Measures. Oral antibiotic Rx _____*(MIS)
                                                    or
alternative antibiotic Rx _____*(MIS).

Consider OTC or Rx antibacterial soap _____*(MIS).

Physician Consultation. Consider for facial and particularly periorbital involvement, genital/rectal involvement, systemic symptomatology, any underlying predisposing conditions all children under 3 months.

Referral.

Immediate Transfer.

Follow-up Plan. Recheck in _____ days if not improved, sooner if worse.

	Initials	Date
Physician		
ARNP		

* unless allergic, containdicated
or pregnant/lactating

Herpes Simplex Type I
Primary and Recurrent
Child and Adult

EVALUATION/DIAGNOSTIC PROTOCOL

Subjective

History. Primary symptoms (generalized mouth soreness, high fevers, irritability, avoidance of eating and drinking). Recurrent (symptoms course).

Objective

Physical Examination. Primary. General appearance, vital signs, complete ENT exam, neck exam (note that eruption may occur anywhere on the skin or on any mucus membranes). If other than the oral pharynx, then regional lymphoreticular examination and complete skin exam. Recurrent. ENT exam, neck exam.

Lab. Viral (herpes) cultures or herpes titers (acute and convalescent) may be indicated (depends on personal patient apprehension and/or social climate)

Assess severity of primary infection, in particular in children as it affects oral intake. **Differential Diagnosis.** HSV-II, viruses causing herpangina, varicella-zoster. **Complications.** Ophthalmic involvement and erythema multiforme.

PLAN/MANAGEMENT PROTOCOL

General Measures. Primary and secondary infection: Explain to patient or parents that the primary infection and its symptoms lasts 5 to 10 days but that viral shedding may continue from 2 to 6 weeks.

Explain that most HSV-I infections are subclinical, consequently it can have been contracted from a source unaware of actual infection.

Encourage plenty of neutral foods and fluids (breast milk, formula, milkshakes, ice cream). Avoid citrus, fruits, acidy juices and spicy foods. Recommend dose of acetaminophen for age and weight.

Follow good oral and general hygienic measures.

Specific Measures.

Primary: consider Rx _____ *(MIS).

Recurrent: consider topical Rx _____ *(MIS)
                                    or
consider oral Rx _____ *(MIS).

Physician Consultation. Consider for severe primary infection, referral or conjunctivitis or keratitis.

Referral.

Immediate Transfer.

Follow-up Plan. Recheck if not resolved in _____ days, sooner if worse. Consider convalescent titer (_____ weeks).

	Initials	Date
* unless allergic, containdicated	Physician	
or pregnant/lactating	ARNP	

Cutaneous larva migrans

EVALUATION/DIAGNOSTIC PROTOCOL
Subjective
History. Must have history of possible exposure to cat or dog hookworms.

Objective
Physical Examination. Complete skin exam (typically, serpiginous erythematous rash, hence the name "creeping eruption").

Lab. Usually not necessary.

Assess severity. **Differential Diagnosis.** Impetigo, contact dermatitis, and dermatophytes. **Complications.** Excoriations and secondary infection.

PLAN/MANAGEMENT PROTOCOL
General Measures.
Instruct parent or patient in how to avoid.

Specific Measures.
Consider oral or topical antihelminthic Rx _____*(MIS).

Consider oral antihistamine OTC/Rx _____*(MIS).

Physician Consultation. Consider if diagnostic doubt.

Referral.

Immediate Transfer.

Follow-up Plan. Recheck if not resolved in _____ week(s).

	Initials	Date
* unless allergic, containdicated or pregnant/lactating	Physician ARNP	

Scabies

EVALUATION/DIAGNOSTIC PROTOCOL
Subjective
History. Describe onset of rash and its course. Pattern of pruritis. Possible exposure. Last menstrual period.

Objective
Physical Examination. Skin for erythematous macules and papules, often with a characteristic burrow. Rarely the mite appears as a black dot in a small vesicle. Lesions often excoriated. Location: Interdigital webs of hands or feet, wrist creases, nipples, umbilicus, genitalia, buttocks and gluteal cleft.

Lab. Scrape lesion, look for mite parts or mite feces after placing drop of oil on the scrapings. Scan at low power.

Assess severity. **Differential Diagnosis** is confusing, depending on the numbers and locations of the lesions, but includes: pediculosis, pyoderma, atopic dermatitis and neurodermatitis. **Complications**. Secondary infection and often social turmoil.

PLAN/MANAGEMENT PROTOCOL
General Measures. Explain scabies and its mode of transmission. Hot wash all clothes, bedding and linens. Instruct parent or patient that itching may persist 5 to 14 days after successful treatment.

Specific Measures.
Consider oral antihistamine OTC or Rx _____ *(MIS).

For those over 3 years, give Rx for gammabenzine hexachloride _____.
Instruct in usage with cautions *(MIS)
or

as an alternative crotamiton 10% cream _____ *(MIS).

Physician Consultation. Consider for children under 3, severe infestation, repeated failure to respond to therapy.

Referral.

Follow-up Plan. Consider reapplication in one week if treatment failure. Follow-up at any time for signs or symptoms of secondary skin infection or adverse drug reaction.

	Initials	Date
* unless allergic, containdicated	Physician	
or pregnant/lactating	ARNP	

Dermatophilis pentrans
Chiggers

EVALUATION/DIAGNOSTIC PROTOCOL

Subjective

History. History of exposure to grasses and shrubs that may have harbored the mites.

Objective

Physical Examination. Complete examination of skin with attention to areas that have been covered by clothing, in particular by underwear.

Lab.

Assess severity. **Differential Diagnosis.** Insect bites/stings, scabies, varicella. **Complications.** Excoriations and secondary infections.

PLAN/MANAGEMENT PROTOCOL

General Measures. Dispel myths, these are bites. Ice water compressing or gentle ice massage may help with itching.

It is most important to emphasize prevention of future skin contact with the mites. This can be achieved by wearing long-sleeved shirts, long pants, and boots, and taping the clothing at the ankles, wrists, and waist, and dusting these areas with flowers of sulfur powder or by using an insect repellent. Wash the clothing immediately after exposure and shower well.

Specific Measures.
Consider oral OTC/Rx antihistamine _____ *(MIS).

Physician Consultation. Consider for diagnostic uncertainty.

Referral.

Immediate Transfer. Usually not necessary.

Follow-up Plan. Usually not necessary.

	Initials	Date
* unless allergic, containdicated	Physician	
or pregnant/lactating	ARNP	

Pediculosis Capitis

EVALUATION/DIAGNOSTIC PROTOCOL
<u>Subjective</u>
History. Course of itching and history of known exposure.

<u>Objective</u>
Physical Examination. Lice are difficult to find. Look for nits in the hair behind the ears and on the posterior scalp.

Lab.

<u>Assess</u> severity. **Differential Diagnosis** includes other scalp dermatoses such as seborrhea, impetigo, neurodermatitis and tinea capitis. **Complications.** Excoriations, secondary infection, and reactive adenopathy.

<u>PLAN</u>/MANAGEMENT PROTOCOL
General Measures. Emphasize ease of transmission as eggs can survive for days without human contact.

Remove nits with fine-tooth comb (usually after therapy).

All bedding, clothes, combs and brushes must be hot washed the day of treatment, some furniture may require spraying.

Specific Measures.
For those over 3 years, consider gammabenzine hexachloride shampoo _____*(MIS)
                                               or
pyrethrin for everybody (including young children and pregnant women if absolutely necessary) _____*(MIS).

Physician Consultation. Consider for children under 3 and pregnant women, therapeutic failure.

Referral.

Immediate Transfer.

Follow-up Plan. For therapeutic failure or recurrence.

	Initials	Date
* unless allergic, containdicated or pregnant/lactating	Physician ARNP	

Tinea Corporis

EVALUATION/DIAGNOSTIC PROTOCOL

Subjective

History. Onset and course of the rash and other symptoms (little or no itching at the site).

Objective

Physical Examination. Initially erythematous papule or macule which enlarges. As this happens the central area clears, leaving a reddened raised scaly rim around a more normal appearing center located most commonly on exposed body surfaces.

Lab. Scrape the border and do a KOH microscopic exam.

Assessment is directed at the **Differential Diagnosis**, which is vast and includes atopic, contact and seborrheic dermatoses as well as psoriasis, pityriasis rosea and neurodermatitis. **Complications**. Secondary infections.

PLAN/MANAGEMENT PROTOCOL

General Measures. Explain to patient that even though this is often called "ringworm," it is a fungus. Wash with soap and water, then apply recommended medication.

Specific Measures. Topical anti-fungal OTC or Rx _____*(MIS).

Physician Consultation. Consider if severe or treatment failure.

Referral.

Immediate Transfer.

Follow-up Plan. _____ weeks if not completely cleared.

		Initials	Date
* unless allergic, containdicated	Physician		
or pregnant/lactating	ARNP		

Tinea Cruris

EVALUATION/DIAGNOSTIC PROTOCOL

Subjective

History. Onset and course of symptoms. Any aggravating (recent hot weather, history of other circumstances that promote friction or maceration) or alleviating factors?

Objective

Physical Examination. Complete skin examination. Note this is often associated with tinea pedis.

Lab. Scrape the border of the lesion to do a KOH microscopic examination or consider culture.

Assessment is directed at the **Differential Diagnosis**, which is vast and includes atopic, contact and seborrheic dermatitis as well as psoriasis, neurodermatitis, erythrasma and especially candida. **Complications** could include candida.

PLAN/MANAGEMENT PROTOCOL

General Measures. Discuss measures to keep the groin dry by powdering after bathing and changing underwear frequently.

Specific Measures.
Treat with OTC/Rx topical antifungal _____*(MIS)
                                              or
combination antifungal/corticosteroid _____*(MIS).

Physician Consultation. Usually not necessary.

Referral. Per attending.

Immediate Transfer. Usually not necessary.

Follow-up Plan. Recheck in _____ weeks if not completely cleared.

Initials   Date

* unless allergic, containdicated   Physician
  or pregnant/lactating   ARNP

Tinea Pedis

EVALUATION/DIAGNOSTIC PROTOCOL
Subjective
History. Onset and course of symptoms. Any history of circumstances that promote moisture/maceration? Any previous treatment?

Objective
Physical Examination. Complete skin exam.

Lab. Consider scraping the active margins of the involved area to do a KOH microscopic exam or a fungal culture.

Assessment/Differential Diagnosis/Complications. It is often difficult to assess and differentiate from candida or just maceration/intertrigo, which obviously can be concomitant.

PLAN/MANAGEMENT PROTOCOL
General Measures. Wash feet several times a day with soap and water, paying particular attention to clean between the toes. The feet should be dried thoroughly. Foot powder or absorbing cotton socks help to keep feet dry. Consider changing socks frequently. Less moisture accumulates in sandals or canvas sneakers than in enclosed shoes or more elaborate track wear. Put on socks before underwear to avoid getting tinea cruris.

Specific Measures
Consider topical OTC/Rx antifungal _____*(MIS)
                                                        or
with consultant approval oral antifungal Rx _____*(MIS).

Physician Consultation. For diagnostic uncertainty or treatment failure.

Referral.

Immediate Transfer.

Follow-up Plan. Every _____months (or as necessary if oral therapy started).

	Initials	Date
Physician		
ARNP		

* unless allergic, containdicated
or pregnant/lactating

Tinea Versicolor

EVALUATION/DIAGNOSTIC PROTOCOL
Subjective
History. Skin history focusing on course and location of lesions. Note that these patches in the summer in sun-exposed areas do not tan and thus appear lighter than surrounding skin. In the winter the patches appear darker. Rarely is there itching.

Objective
Physical Examination. Complete skin exam. Lesions are located mainly on the upper trunk, consist of small, large, or confluent patches which shed a fine scale when scratched lightly.

Lab. Scrape lesions, do a KOH prep.

Assessment is directed at the **Differential Diagnosis**, which includes atopic dermatitis, seborrheic dermatisis, vitiligo, pityriasis rosea. (See those sections.) **Complications**. None.

PLAN/MANAGEMENT PROTOCOL
General Measures. Alert the patient that recurrence is very common, but that this is always a benign condition.

Specific Measures. Treat topically with _____*(MIS)

or

alternative Rx _____*(MIS).

Physician Consultation. Consider for diagnostic uncertainty or treatment failure.

Referral.

Immediate Transfer. Usually not necessary.

Follow-up Plan. Recheck in _____ weeks if not improved/resolved.

Initials   Date

* unless allergic, containdicated   Physician
or pregnant/lactating   ARNP

Molluscum Contagiosum

EVALUATION/DIAGNOSTIC PROTOCOL
<u>Subjective</u>
History. Lesions only symptomatic because of location or unsightliness.

<u>Objective</u>
Physical Examination. Complete skin exam. The lesions classically are flesh-colored to pearly white raised papules with central umbilicated papules.

Lab. Consider biopsy if diagnosis in doubt.

<u>Assess</u> severity in terms of number and also location. **Differential Diagnosis.** Warts. **Complications.** Secondary infection.

PLAN/MANAGEMENT PROTOCOL
General Measures. Consider not treating if minimal lesions as this disorder can resolve spontaneously.

Specific Measures. Apply _____*(MIS)

or consider destruction by cryotherapy or electrodessication.

Physician Consultation. Consider for severity.

Referral.

Immediate Transfer. Not necessary.

Follow-up Plan. Re-examination necessary if lesions become symptomatic or if marked increase in number, or if no significant response to therapy.

	Initials	Date
* unless allergic, containdicated	Physician	
or pregnant/lactating	ARNP	

Warts

EVALUATION/DIAGNOSTIC PROTOCOL

<u>Subjective</u>

History.   Symptomatic because of location or unsightliness and course.

<u>Objective</u>

Physical Examination.   Flesh-colored hyperkeratotic raised lesions with characteristic black flecks centrally.

Lab.   None.

<u>Assess</u> severity by number, size, location and degree of disturbance to the patient. **Differential Diagnosis.** Molluscum. **Complications.** Secondary infection, unsightly, and uncomfortable in certain locations.

PLAN/MANAGEMENT PROTOCOL

General Measures.   None.

Specific Measures.   Apply to common warts _____*(MIS)

                                                                                        or

apply to common warts _____*(MIS).

Pare plantar warts

                                                            and/or

apply OTC or Rx keratolytic.

Physician Consultation. Consider for unusually located, numerous warts, exceedingly large warts.

Referral.

Immediate Transfer.

Follow-up Plan. Dictated by the modality of therapy but should be sooner if signs of secondary infection occur after treatment.

	Initials	Date
* unless allergic, containdicated or pregnant/lactating	Physician ARNP	

CHAPTER 12
NEUROLOGY

<u>Tension Headaches</u>

EVALUATION/DIAGNOSTIC PROTOCOL
<u>Subjective</u>
History. General, headache description, location, quality, aggravating alleviating factors, accompanying symptomatology.

<u>Objective</u>
Physical Examination. General appearance, vital signs, head, ENT, neck, complete neurologic.

Lab. None.

<u>Assess</u> severity. **Differentiate** tension from other common causes, including the various migraines, cluster headaches, sinusitis, and the rare but serious causes, including subarachnoid bleed, meningitis, encephalitis, CVA, brain tumor. **Complications** are related to the patient's stress be it mechanical or emotional.

<u>PLAN/MANAGEMENT PROTOCOL</u>
General Measures. Reassurance, taking time to explain muscle contraction. Relaxation techniques and massage.

Specific Measures.
OTC or Rx analgesic _____*(MIS).

Author's Note: With children, controlled substance use should be avoided. Instead employ non-drug therapy.

Consider limited Rx for narcotic analgesic _____*(MIS)

or

consider Rx for mild muscle relaxant/tranquilizer _____*(MIS).

Physician Consultation. Consider for severity, unclear diagnosis, peculiar symptomatology.

Referral.

Immediate Transfer.

Follow-up Plan. In _____ weeks or sooner if worse.

Initials   Date

* unless allergic, contraindicated   Physician
pregnant/lactating   ARNP

Migraine Headaches

EVALUATION/DIAGNOSTIC PROTOCOL
Subjective
History. General, headache description, location, quality, prodrome (aura) and timing, aggravating (meals and specific foods) or alleviating factors, accompanying symptomatology. Family history of migraine. Complete medication history OTC/Rx/ illicit. Any relationship to menses?

Objective
Physical Examination. General appearance, vital signs, head, ENT, neck, complete neurologic.

Lab.

Assess type of migraine: classic from common from mixed and variant type (though different in character, cluster headaches may have similar origin). Differential Diagnosis. Tension from other common causes, including the various migraines, cluster headaches, sinusitis, and the rare but serious causes, including subarachnoid bleed, meningitis, encephalitis, CVA, brain tumor. Complications. Usually none.

PLAN/MANAGEMENT PROTOCOL
General Measures. Explain the nature of migraines, in particular avoiding known personal precipitants, stressors, foods, etc. Provide or recommend reinforcing educational literature (such as Headache by Consumer Reports). Emphasize regular exercise and stress reduction/relaxation techniques.

Specific Measures.
FOR PRODROME OR EARLY ACUTE PHASE, immediately
Give dose of _____*(MIS)
                                          or
give Rx for _____*(MIS).

FOR LATE ACUTE PHASE the above abortive agents don't usually help, therefore
Consider Rx oral narcotic analgesic (IF NO VOMITING) _____*(MIS)

                                          or
IF VOMITING, give IM narcotic analgesic/antinauseant combination _____
_____*(MIS).

Subsequently, institute prophylactic therapy with
beta blocker Rx _____*(MIS),

or an antidepressant Rx _____*(MIS),

or a calcium agonist Rx _____*(MIS).

Physician Consultation. Consider when making initial diagnosis of migraines or for severity, therapeutic failure, persistent symptomatology.

Referral.

Immediate Transfer.

Follow-up Plan. Recheck in _____ weeks or as appropriate.

                                                          Initials   Date

* unless allergic, contraindicated   Physician
pregnant/lactating   ARNP

Acute Vertigo

EVALUATION/DIAGNOSTIC PROTOCOL

Subjective

History. Should be carefully obtained including the patient's description. Often, the patient must be coaxed beyond the term "dizziness" to be certain the problem is vertigo and not presyncope. Any associated symptoms? Aggravating and alleviating factors, predisposing circumstances, and underlying conditions. Review drug use OTC/Rx/illicit. LMP. Emergency consultation if sudden onset or accompanying headache.

Objective

Physical Examination. General appearance, vital signs (any orthostasis?), complete ENT, complete cardiovascular and complete neurologic exams (note maneuvers that alleviate symptoms)

Lab. CBC, glucose and other tests as indicated.

Assessment is directed at differentiating the benign causes from the serious causes of vertigo and from presyncope/orthostasis and its etiologies. **Differential Diagnosis** includes labyrinthitis, benign positional vertigo, migraine variant, Meniere's syndrome, drug side effects, hyperventilation and vasovagal syncope, other causes of orthostasis (severe anemia/bleed), hypoglycemia, cerebellar or brainstem tumor/stroke/hemorrhage. **Complications** depend on the etiology, but even the self-limited causes significantly affect perception and steadiness consequently increasing the risk of injury.

PLAN/MANAGEMENT PROTOCOL

General Measures. Explain to the patient and family the difficulty in diagnosing the etiology of a vertigo and the seriousness of some causes. If certain this is a benign cause, then outline the course and measures the patient can follow to prevent self-injury. Hyperventilators should be taught rebreathing (paper bag) and relaxation techniques. Review signs or symptoms that require immediate follow-up including: intractable vomiting, persistent or worsening vertigo, persistent or severe headache.

Specific Measures.
Consider symptomatic relief with Rx for meclizine_____*(MIS)
                                    or
alternative Rx _____*(MIS).

Physician Consultation. Consider as necessary in all cases.

Referral. As indicated to neurologist.

Immediate Transfer. For those suspected of serious intracranial event/pathology.

Follow-up Plan. Must be individualized.

	Initials	Date
* unless allergic, contraindicated	Physician	
pregnant/lactating	ARNP	

Parkinson's Disease

EVALUATION/DIAGNOSTIC PROTOCOL

Subjective

History. Onset and progression of symptoms with attention to description of tremor (abolished by sleep or intentional movement of limb, usually begins in one hand, spreads to ipsilateral foot), possible postural tremor, "cogwheel" or ratchet type rigidity, bradykinesia, change in posture (flexed). Complete medical history, family history, medication history--OTC and prescription. Social history and support network.

Objective

Physical Examination. Vital signs. Complete medical exam with attention to neurological exam, including a mental status exam.

Lab. CBC, electrolytes, thyroid profile, consider drug screens, CT or MRI scans, EEG, or spinal tap or _____.

Assess whether this is secondary parkinsonism or idiopathic Parkinson's disease, or another hypokinetic disorder; if diagnosis made by neurologist, assess patient's level of functioning, medical, social and rehabilatative needs. **Differential Diagnosis.** Hypo/hyperthyroidism, depression with psychomotor retardation, benign essential tremor, medication side effects, alcohol withdrawal, encephalitis, head trauma, hydrocephalus, exposure to toxic chemicals, Alzheimer's or Huntington's disease. **Complications.** Progression of disease causing decline in patient's functioning ability (physical and mental) especially if not treated by medication.

PLAN/MANAGEMENT PROTOCOL

General Measures. Extensive support is crucial to assist patient and family in dealing with the physical and mental changes. Physical therapy referrals and Parkinson support group referrals should be made and followed up on. Assess family needs and coping skills periodically; be alert to signs of depression. Educate patient and family about meds and potential side effects of treatment. Provide or recommend reinforcing educational material (such as Parkinson's Handbook from Cunsomer Reports).

Specific Measures. (Usually prescribed by neurologist.)
Consider _____
_____
_____

Physician Consultation. Generally, on all suspected cases; on follow-up visits as indicated.

Referral. Usually refer to neurologist for consult/definitive diagnosis. Alternatively, _____.

Follow-up Plan. Until diagnosis is established, every _____ days/weeks. Once diagnosis is established co-ordinate follow-up with stage of disease, physical therapist/neurologist consultations and patient or family needs, usually every _____ months.

		Initials	Date
* unless allergic, contraindicated	Physician		
pregnant/lactating	ARNP		

Alzheimer's Disease

EVALUATION/DIAGNOSTIC PROTOCOL

Subjective

History. Current medical history (onset and course of dementia and any concurrent other symptoms). Complete medical history, family history (any first degree relatives with dementia), social history with focus on support network, review of systems. Comprehensive drug use history OTC, prescription and illicit. Occupational and exposure history.

Objective

Physical Examination. Vital signs, complete physical exam with a comprehensive neurologic exam (decreased visuospatial skills) including a mental status exam (memory loss and anomia characteristic but not definitive). Note: The authors strongly recommend the use of a standardized testing instrument such as Mini-Mental Status Exam (reproduced on page 16-20 by permission of Pergamon Press) and also formal psychometric evaluation.

Lab. CBC, chemistry panel, thyroid profile (include TSH), ESR, B12, folate, RPR, urinalysis. Consider urine drug screen, EEG, CT or MRI of brain.

Assessment is very difficult because of the variability of early Alzheimer's and consequently is directed at distinguishing from the other **Differential Diagnostic** considerations. The most common treatable dementias should not be missed. These include pseudodementia of major depression, drug induced cognitive impairment, and multi-infarct dementia. Other causes include vascular disorders, space-occupying lesions, metabolic and nutritional causes, infections, toxic effects, other specific neurologic syndromes. **Complications.** Progression of disease causing decline in patient's functioning ability (physical and mental) especially if not treated by medication.

PLAN/MANAGEMENT PROTOCOL

General Measures. Therapy is directed at support for the patient and family. A functional rating system for activities of daily living will be very helpful in making practical suggestions and in re-evaluating for increasing needs. They should be made aware that this is the cause of over 50% of dementia and that the cause is unknown. Provide or recommend educational materials. Also, encourage joining a support group (Alzheimer's Association, 1-800-621-0379).

Specific Measures. Though there is no specific therapy, some feel there is value in using metabolic enhancers and vasodilators. Specific therapeutic agents may be needed for delusions or hallucinations, aggressive behaviors, depression, sleep difficulties, and agitation.

Physician Consultation. Generally on all suspected cases and at apparent conclusion of initial evaluation. On follow-up visits as indicated.

Referral. Usually refer to neurologist for current/definitive diagnosis.

Follow-up Plan. Until diagnosis is established, every _____ days/weeks. Once diagnosis is established co-ordinate follow-up with stage of disease, physical therapist/neurologist consultations and patient or family needs, usually every _____ months.

Initials   Date

* unless allergic, contraindicated   Physician
pregnant/lactating   ARNP

CHAPTER 13
ENDOCRINOLOGY, METABOLIC DISORDERS AND NUTRITION

Obesity

EVALUATION/DIAGNOSTIC PROTOCOL
<u>Subjective</u>
History. Past attempts at weight reduction, familial obesity, length of time overweight, psychological factors related to obesity, current diet diary, past medical history, exercise history.

<u>Objective</u>
Physical Examination. Weight, vital signs, complete P/E as indicated.

Lab. As indicated--consider lipid profile, TSH, uric acid, _____ and/or _____.

<u>Assessment</u>. Determine percentage above ideal body weight--greater than 30% indicates obesity. Assess motivation and/or underlying psychological factors that hinder successful weight reduction. **Differential Diagnosis**. Primary hypothyroidism, Cushing's syndrome. **Complications** include hypertension, cardiovascular disease, diabetes, arthritis, and kidney disease.

PLAN/MANAGEMENT PROTOCOL
General Measures. Emphasize importance of lifestyle modification versus short-term fad diets for long-term success. Teach behavior modification techniques and have patient keep a diary of food intake, mood, time, and other related data if appropriate. Individualize teaching program and give psychological support. Try to involve other family members. Consider referral to weight loss support group and/or professional counseling to deal with body image. Insist on program of regular physical activity.

Specific Measures. The authors do not recommend drug therapy as an approach.

Physician Consultation. With suspicion of underlying pathology or with development of complications.

Referral. To local supportive programs. For professional counseling as appropriate. Pending physician consultation, a medically supervised fast may be utilized if available in your community.

Immediate Transfer.

Follow-up Plan. During initial teaching and counseling, every _____, then follow up every _____.

<u>Hyperlipoproteinemia a/k Hyperlipidemia</u>
<u>Adults</u>

<u>EVALUATION/DIAGNOSTIC PROTOCOL</u>
<u>Subjective</u>
History. Specific emphasis should be on nutritional history and personal or family history of hyperlipidemia. (There are no symptoms.)

<u>Objective</u>
Physical Examination. When opportunity permits, a complete physical examination should be performed.

Lab. Diagnosis requires laboratory testing. Sufficient preliminary screening includes a fasting cholesterol and triglycerides. More accurate diagnosis follows obtaining a complete fasting lipid profile, including cholesterol (and paralleling low density lipoprotein), triglycerides (and paralleling very low density lipoprotein), high density lipoprotein. Further evaluation should include screening for hypothyroidism (see <u>Hypothyroidism</u>) and diabetes mellitus (see <u>Diabetes Mellitus</u>).

<u>Assess</u> severity, depending on the normal ranges for your laboratory. Briefly, the upper limit of normal for cholesterol is 200 mg/dl and for LDL is 130 mg/dl. The upper limit of normal for triglycerides is 250 mg/dl. HDL less than 35 mg/dl is a risk factor on its own. The implications of this problem relate to other cardiovascular risk factors. However, the most useful indicator may be the ratio of LDL/HDL (3.0, preferably 2.0). **Differential Diagnosis** is amongst the primary and secondary hyperlipidemias. **Complications** vary from localized lipid deposits to pancreatitis to the gamut of atherosclerotic vascular disorders.

<u>PLAN/MANAGEMENT PROTOCOL</u>
General Measures. Patient should be educated in the nature of the problem as it might affect longevity. Similarly, they should be helped to understand the implications of dietary fat intake, and beyond that even total caloric intake, explaining how this in part is balanced against level of exercise. **Habit modification must be emphasized and reemphasized**. Give reinforcing educational materials (such as those from the American Heart Assoc.) and involve family members in educational sessions. Individualize a regular exercise program. Consider screening other family members.

Specific Measures. Consider physician consultation.
Consider an Rx for a bile acid sequestrant _____ *(MIS)
                                        or
as alternative, HMG CoA reductase inhibitor _____ *(MIS).

For hypertriglyceridemia, consider an Rx for _____ *(MIS).

Physician Consultation. Consider for any patient who has a lipid value more than 1½ times the high normal or L/H > 4.0, target organ involvement, or requiring drug therapy.

Referral. For complications as indicated. Consider a nutritionist, too.

Follow-up Plan. Individualzed rechecks _____ week(s) to reinforce habit changes. Repeat lipid survey every _____ months. Drugs will require additional follow up.

                                                          Initials   Date
* unless allergic, contraindicated   Physician
or pregnant/lactating   ARNP

Diabetes Mellitus, Initial Visit

EVALUATION/DIAGNOSTIC PROTOCOL

Subjective

History. Signs and symptoms--onset and progression, past medical history, drug history, family history.

Objective

Physical Examination. Weight, vital signs. Diagnosis determined by lab findings. Complete PE with particular attention to skin, eye, neuro, and cardiovascular exam should always be performed on newly-diagnosed diabetic.

Lab. Urine dip or UA but not adequate for diagnosis. Symptomatic patients: plasma glucose above 200 is diagnostic. Asymptomatic patients: fasting plasma glucose above 140 on more than one occasion. If unable to establish diagnosis, then do GTT. Plasma glucose of 200 mg or higher at 2 hours is diagnostic of diabetes. Consider Hbg AIC chemistry panel, thyroid panel, EKG, and chest x-ray.

Assessment. Determine severity of disease, whether it is insulin-dependent or non-insulin-dependent and factors contributing to condition. **Differential Diagnosis** includes transient effects of drugs or chemicals, pancreatic disease, other endocrine disease and less common causes. **Complications** include hyperglycemic exacerbations and/or ketoacidosis, hypoglycemia, vascular disease including retinopathy and nephropathy, skin infections, UTIs and monilial infections.

PLAN/MANAGEMENT PROTOCOL

General Measures. Therapy is based on comprehensive patient and family education since patient, to a large degree, assists in managing therapy. The relationship of diet, physical activity and medications must be conveyed in printed information as well as referrals to community support group must be supplied. (See follow-up sections for specific IDDM or NIDDM patients).

Specific Measures. See IDDM and NIDDM sections.

Physician Consultation. Consider on all newly-diagnosed diabetics and all abnormal glucose levels or on undiagnosed patients.

Referral. Consider consultation with endocrinologist on newly-diagnosed diabetics if IDDM is suspected, particularly if under 40. Consider consultation on other diagnosed adult-onset patients or as complications arise as appropriate. Ophthalmologist consult as indicated.

Immediate Transfer. With suspicion of ketoacidosis.

Follow-up Plan. Will vary depending on type. During establishment of diagnosis office visit frequency should be individualized _____.

Initials   Date

* unless allergic, contraindicated   Physician
or pregnant/lactating   ARNP

Diabetes Mellitus, Follow-Up Visit,
Non-insulin-Dependent

EVALUATION/DIAGNOSTIC PROTOCOL

Subjective

History. Review of symptoms, patient's acceptance level and compliance with therapeutic regimen. If on drug therapy ask about side effects, hypoglycemia, and review home monitoring charts.

Objective

Physical Examination. Vital signs, skin, neuro, cardiac and vascular exams at each visit or complete PE yearly as indicated by severity and course of disease.

Lab. Plasma glucose measurements or glucose oxidase reagent strip measurements of whole blood if home monitoring shows unacceptably levels or every _____ months routinely. Glycosylated hemoglobin (Hbg AIC) measurements as indicated. UA every _____ or as indicated. CBC and chem panel every _____. Consider EKG, chest x-ray, creatinine clearance.

Assessment. Adequacy of blood glucose levels, patient compliance with weight loss program, and status of co-existing conditions such as cardiovascular disease, depression. Complications. Same as for IDDM.

PLAN/MANAGEMENT PROTOCOL

General Measures. Patient education for most adult onset in IDDM patients, the cornerstone of therapy is weight reduction. Visits should be frequent and include spouse or significant other, especially during initial sessions. Total caloric intake must be individualized to body weight and height of patient. Plan daily exercise program. Urine and/or self blood glucose monitoring.

Specific Measures. Consider oral hypoglycemic drugs may be used in conjunction with dietary therapy. Dosage should begin low with gradual increases.

Rx _____ *(MIS)

or

Rx _____ *(MIS).

Endogenous insulin may be needed. See Insulin Use protocol for IDDM.

Physician Consultation. Consider when significant problems with compliance or poor blood glucose control, medication side effects, development of secondary microvascular complications.

Referral. Consider if acceptable blood glucose control is not achieved; consider nutritionist or dietitian as indicated.

Immediate Transfer. Severe hypoglycemia.

Follow-up Plan. Every _____ until diet program is effectively underway, and then every _____.

	Initials	Date

* unless allergic, contraindicated
or pregnant/lactating

Physician
ARNP

Diabetes Mellitus, Follow-Up Visit, Insulin-Dependent

EVALUATION/DIAGNOSTIC PROTOCOL

Subjective

History. Assess impact of illness on individual and families' functioning and emotional health, needs for further education, review of symptoms, medication side effects, diet diary, exercise regimen, compliance with management plan, and review of home monitoring charts.

Objective

Physical Examination. Every _____, vital signs, weight, fundoscopic, skin, neuro, and cardiovascular exam. Every _____, complete PE.

Lab. On newly-diagnosed patients, hospitalization often necessary to fine-tune insulin control. Once under acceptable control, FBS and glycosylated hemoglobin (Hgb AIC) every _____. CBC and chem panel or _____ tests every _____. UAs every _____.

Assessment. Adequacy of plasma glucose control, reduction of risk factors, and adjustment of patient to treatment regimen. **Complications.** Inability of patient to properly administer insulin, psychological difficulties in coping with disease, hypoglycemic episodes including insulin shock, ketoacidosis, or diabetic coma (see Initial Visit, Complications).

PLAN/MANAGEMENT PROTOCOL

General Measures. Coordinate teaching plan with endocrinologist or with hospital health educator as indicated and include family member(s). Dietary modification in accordance with presence of obesity and concurrent medical therapy. Emphasize consistent dietary pattern with attention to composition and timing of meals. Exchange lists can assist patient to maintain consistency of carbohydrate levels and calories while still enjoying freedom of choice. Composition: carbohydrate (60-65%), protein (10-20%), fat (25-35%). Encourage high fiber content. Limit or avoid alcohol use, which predisposes to hypoglycemia as well as affects sulfonylurea metabolism. Medication teaching: Coordinate with hospital or endocrinologist. Include proper technique, side effects—especially how to recognize and treat hypoglycemia. Daily exercise program—individualized and coordinated with meal timing and insulin administration. Teach travel considerations.

Specific Measures. Prescribing insulin dosage with therapeutic adjustment should be made with physician consultation. Use the following lines for comments or guidelines for instituting and adjusting insulin dosage.

_____
_____
_____

Physician Consultation. Consider for difficulties with patient compliance, signs of infection or secondary complications, see preceding section.

Referral. Ophthalmologist evaluation every _____. Podiatry referral as indicated. Dental referral as indicated.

Immediate Transfer. See previous section.

Follow-up Plan. Office visit every _____ after initial diagnosis and teaching sessions complete. Follow-up at first signs of infection or if poor control detected by patient's home monitoring.

	Initials	Date
* unless allergic, contraindicated or pregnant/lactating	Physician ARNP	

Hypothyroidism

EVALUATION/DIAGNOSTIC PROTOCOL

Subjective

History. Complete review of system (with attention focused on recent weight change, energy level, sleep habits, cold intolerance). In addition, patient may complain of dry skin, hoarseness, constipation, and menstrual irregularity. Is there a family history of thyroid disease? Review both over-the-counter and prescription medication.

Objective

Physical Examination. Complete physical examination is necessary (signs may be subtle and include increased weight, decreased pulse, hair loss, dry skin, slow recovery phase of Achilles tendon reflex).

Lab. Total T4, T3 uptake, TSH (consider TRH or challenge after consultation).

Assessment is directed at determining severity of hypothyroidism. If not severe, replacement can be phased in gradually. **Differential Diagnosis.** Nephrotic syndrome. **Complications** include hypotension, bradycardia, hypoventilation, hypothermia, and ultimately myxedema coma. Fluid and electrolyte imbalance are frequent concomitants.

PLAN/MANAGEMENT PROTOCOL

General Measures. Explain to the patient the function of the thyroid gland and the importance of treating impaired function.

Specific Measures. When the diagnosis is certain, begin thyroid replacement with _____*(MIS).

Physician Consultation. Consider for all patients with proven hypothyroidism.

Referral.

Immediate Transfer.

Follow-up Plan. Follow up in _____ weeks to be preceded by repeat thyroid function panel, including TSH.

		Initials	Date
* unless allergic, contraindicated or pregnant/lactating	Physician ARNP		

Hyperthyroidism

EVALUATION/DIAGNOSTIC PROTOCOL
<u>Subjective</u>
History. General history and review of systems (weight loss, palpitations, agitation, tremulousness, heat intolerance, significant emotional instability). Family history of thyroid disease. Prescription and non-prescription medications.

<u>Objective</u>
Physical Examination. Complete physical exam (weight loss, tachycardia, hypertension, fine tremor).

Lab. Total T4, T3 uptake (consider T3 by RIA), thyroid scan and R131 uptake after consultation with attending.

Assess severity of thyrotoxicosis. **Differential Diagnosis**. Distinguish the different causes of hyperthyroidism, including Graves' disease, toxic multinodular goiter, hyperfunctioning adenomas, thyroid carcinomas. **Complications** include cardiac arrhythmia, congestive heart failure, seizures, psychosis, and ultimately thyroid storm.

PLAN/MANAGEMENT PROTOCOL
General Measures. Explain nature of thyroid function, relating it to the patient's symptomatology of hyperfunction. More significantly, caution about signs and symptoms of thyroid storm.

Specific Measures. Ultimately directed at the etiology of a patient's thyroid toxicosis.

Consider prescribing beta blocker _____*(MIS).

Physician Consultation. On all cases of hyperthyroidism, unmedicated yet marked hyperthyroidism.

Referral.

Immediate Transfer. If impending thyroid storm.

Follow-up Plan. Must be individualized.

Initials   Date

* unless allergic, contraindicated   Physician
  or pregnant/lactating   ARNP

New Thyroid Mass or Enlargement

EVALUATION/DIAGNOSTIC PROTOCOL

<u>Subjective</u>

History. General history and review of systems with particular focus on when the patient became aware of mass or enlargement and whether it causes tracheal compression and or dysphagia. Family history of thyroid disease. Medications, prescription and non-prescription.

<u>Objective</u>

Physical Examination. Preferably complete physical exam should be performed with attention to the thyroid.

Lab. T4, T3 uptake, TSH. For a new mass, a thyroid scan after consultation with physician.

<u>Assess</u> whether this is a solitary nodule or goiter while also assessing thyroid function (see <u>Hypothyroidism</u> or <u>Hyperthyroidism</u>). **Differential Diagnosis** of nodules includes, cysts, adenomas (which can run the gamut of function), carcinoma of different types, and even hematoma. Enlargement can represent any type of goiter. **Complications** depend on the type of nodule or goiter and associated effect on thyroid function.

PLAN/MANAGEMENT PROTOCOL

General Measures. Explain the nature of the thyroid. Discuss relative rarity of malignancy and its implications, but more specifically discuss effects of hyperfunctioning nodules and the need for evaluation and treatment. Have a similar discussion about goiters.

Specific Measures depend upon the type of nodule or goiter.

Physician Consultation. In all instances. Immediately if significant hyper-thyroidism.

Referral.

Immediate Transfer.

Follow-up Plan.

Initials   Date

* unless allergic, contraindicated
or pregnant/lactating

Physician
ARNP

Hyperuricemia and Gout

EVALUATION/DIAGNOSTIC PROTOCOL
Subjective
History. Onset and course of symptoms (aggravating and alleviating factors). General medical history, specifically focused on musculoskeletal history. Family history of gout or hyperuricemia. Medication use prescription or OTC. Habit and dietary history.

Objective
Physical Exam. General appearance, vital signs, musculoskeletal, skin (tophaceous deposits), exams.

Lab. CBC, uric acid, urinalysis. Consider sed rate, ANA, RA latex etc.

Assess severity (asymptomatic hyperuricemia, gouty arthritis acute vs. chronic, or interval phase). Also distinguish primary from secondary. **Differential Diagnosis** other arthridities (including septic joint), pseudogout, sarcoidosis. **Complications** arthritis, tophaceous deposits, nephrolithiasis.

PLAN/MANAGEMENT PROTOCOL
General Measures. Explain the nature of gout. Discuss the myths surrounding this disease. Again, primary gout is inherited. Review high and low purine foods and the need to decrease total purine intake. Encourage plenty of fluids. Give reinforcing educational materials. Consider establishing a contingency plan for acute attacks.

Specific Measures   ACUTE GOUT
Consider Rx for antiinflammatory _____*(MIS)
                                          and/or
Rx for colchicine protocol _____*(MIS)
and consider instituting also

                          MAINTENANCE THERAPY
Long-term Rx for allopurinol _____*(MIS)
                                  and possible
Additional Rx _____*(MIS).

Physician Consultation. Consider for all new cases, diagnostic uncertainty, severe episode, refractory or intolerant to therapy.

Referral.

Immediate Transfer. Usually not necessary.

Follow-up Plan. Recheck in _____day(s) after an acute episode, sooner if worse. Once maintenance is established then follow-up uric acid and visit every _____ months.

	Initials	Date
Physician		
ARNP		

* unless allergic, contraindicated
or pregnant/lactating

Anemia, Iron Deficiency, Children

EVALUATION/DIAGNOSTIC PROTOCOL

Subjective

History. Obtain complete medical history including dietary and neonatal history. Any nutritional supplements? Previous history of anemia or family history?

Objective

Physical Exam. Complete physical exam. Mild anemia is usually asymptomatic.

Lab. Hematocrit is often the first indication of anemia. Consider (either initially or after trial of iron supplementation) a CBC, sickle prep (or hemoglobin electrophoresis), _____, and stool for guaiac and O&P.

Assessment is directed not only at the severity but also at the etiology which includes blood loss either acute or chronic, dietary insufficiency (excessive whole milk in the early years) or inadequate birth supply or newborn hemolytic disease.

	Normal	Hematocrits
2 wks	42-66
3 m-6m	31-41
6 m-6y	33-42
7 y-12	34-40

Differential Diagnosis. Iron deficiency is normochromic normocytic initially, then hypochromic microcytic (which can also be caused by hemoglobinopathies and lead poisoning). The other anemias have other differentials. Complications depend in part on the etiology but as the anemia worsens, increased infections, high output failure and/or failure to thrive.

PLAN/MANAGEMENT PROTOCOL

General Measures. Explain anemia and the need for follow-up. Review appropriate dietary modifications. Set specific guidelines for these changes (for infants being given whole milk resume a commercial formula, for infants on solids encourage the iron-fortified cereals, age appropriate meats, green vegetables, etc. and limit older children to 16 ounces of milk per day). Give educational materials.

Specific Measures.
Recommend or prescribe iron supplementation _____*(MIS).

Physician Consultation. Consider for all infants and for children with hematocrits less than _____, for suspected blood loss, suspected child neglect, or failure for hematocrit to improve after _____ weeks of therapy.

Referral.

Immediate Transfer. With physician consultation or if suspected child neglect.

Follow-up Plan. Repeat hematocrit or _____ in _____ weeks.

Initials   Date

* unless allergic, contraindicated   Physician
or pregnant/lactating   ARNP

Iron Deficiency Anemia, Adults

EVALUATION/DIAGNOSTIC PROTOCOL

Subjective
History. Obtain complete medical history including dietary review. Previous or family history of anemia. Any medications Rx/OTC/illicit? Menstrual change?

Objective
Physical Exam. General appearance, vital signs, abdomen and rectal exams. Ideally a complete physical exam.

Lab. Hematocrit is often the first indication of anemia. In the menstruating female commonly additional testing may be deferred until after a trial of iron supplementation. In a male or subsequently in the female begin with a CBC. The indices direct further testing. Consider percent saturation of transferrin and also _____. Hct in normal males is 42-52 and in females 37-47.

Assessment is directed not only at the severity but at the etiology. **Differential Diagnosis** includes initially the causes of the normochromic normocytic anemias and as anemia worsens, the causes of hypochromic microcytic anemias; blood loss either acute or chronic (menstrual loss is certainly the most common, multigravidas, gastrointestinal loss is not however, that uncommon), dietary insufficiency (due to unusual dietary habits or excessive need for replacement in a frequent blood donor), hemoglobinopathies, hemolytic causes and chronic diseases. The remaining differential is that of the other anemias. **Complications** depend in large part on the etiology but include worsening anemia, infections, high output cardiac failure.

PLAN/MANAGEMENT PROTOCOL
General Measures. Explain anemia and the need for follow-up visits. Review appropriate dietary changes and set specific goals for these changes.

Specific Measures.
Recommend or prescribe iron supplementation _____*(MIS).

Physician Consultation. Consider for patients with hematocrits less than 30, failure to respond to therapy in _____ weeks, evidence of blood loss other than menstrual, severely ill or with orthostasis.

Referral.

Immediate Transfer.

Follow-up Plan. Dictated by the known etiology or working diagnosis. Follow-up hematocrit or _____ in _____ weeks.

	Initials	Date
* unless allergic, contraindicated	Physician	
or pregnant/lactating	ARNP	

Osteoporosis

EVALUATION/DIAGNOSTIC PROTOCOL
Subjective
History. General medical, obstetric, gynecologic, habit (exercise, smoking), diet (calcium intake), family and medication history.

Objective
Physical Exam. Complete physical exam.

Lab. CBC, chemistry panel. Consider bone densitometry.

Assessment is directed at the patient's risk factors, which include inherited factors (family history, slight build/small-boned, fair skin Caucasian or Oriental), nutritional and habit factors (low calcium intake, high caffeine intake, high alcohol use, cigarette smoking, inactivity, high sodium intake), endocrine factors (menopause or premature ovarian failure/removal, diabetes mellitus, hyperthyroidism, Cushing's disease, nulliparity), pharmacologic (steroid use). **Differential Diagnosis**. Osteoarthritis, metastatic carcinoma (multiple myeloma, too), vitamin D deficiency. **Complications**. Fractures, particularly of the hip which carries high mortality within the three months from the time of the occurrence.

PLAN/MANAGEMENT PROTOCOL
General Measures. Educate the patient about their personal risks and the long term consequences. Encourage adequate dietary intake of calcium (at a median level of 1000 mg/day of elemental calcium). Encourage regular exercise. Discourage unhealthful habits. Suggest hormonal therapy, discussing its advantages (modifies menopausal symptomatology; see Menopause) and disadvantages (a minor disadvantage is withdrawal bleeding and a major disadvantage is the increased risk for endometrial carcinoma--even this risk appears to decrease, however, with the addition of a progestogen to the estrogen regime). Provide reinforcing educational literature.

Specific Measures.
Consider calcium supplementation _____*(MIS).

Consider estrogen replacement therapy _____*(MIS)
                                        and
consider progestin added cyclically _____*(MIS).

Physician Consultation. For all patients to be placed on hormonal therapy, who are high risk but are refusing therapy and for those intolerant of therapy/

Referral. For unexpected vaginal bleeding to _____ or
for a fracture to _____.

Follow-up Plan. Recheck in _____ months and thereafter every _____ months.

                                                          Initials   Date

* unless allergic, contraindicated   Physician
or pregnant/lactating   ARNP

CHAPTER 14
PSYCHIATRY

Anxiety

EVALUATION/DIAGNOSTIC PROTOCOL
Subjective
History. Situational psychiatric and situational social history (Why is the patient here now? and What does the patient think is wrong?). Current medical history, past history, family history, family systems diagram, social history, psychiatric history. Current medications: over the counter, prescription and illicit. Other substance use, caffeine, alcohol and tobacco history. other stimulant usage (caffeine), other symptoms.

Objective
Physical Examination. General appearance, vital signs, neurologic exam, mental status exam (observe behavior, appearance, and affect including range and depth, assess mood, observe level of anxiety, explore thought content for obsessessions, phobias, compulsive rituals and suicidal ideations with or without plan of intent) and symptom specific system exam when complete physical exam not possible.

Lab. Usually none but consider broad screening battery, including CBC, chemistry profile and thyroid panel. Strongly consider an MMPI or similar instrument.

Assess presence, degree and source(s) of exogenous stimulus. Assess severity of anxiety and degree of dysfunction and of avoidant behaviors. Assess severity of psycho-social stressors. Assess general functioning. Assess suicide risk. Does this meet DSM III-R criteria? Differential Diagnosis. Drug induced anxiety (caffeine, alcohol, nicotine, amphetamines, sympathomimetic agents, neuroleptic antiemetic agents, monosodium glutamate, and withdrwal phenomenon), medical (hyperthyroidism, hypoglycemia, pheochromocytoma). Complications. More significantly alcoholism, major psychosis, panic disorder, AGITATED DEPRESSION.

PLAN/MANAGEMENT PROTOCOL
General Measures. Conduct the history and physical examination in a non-judgmental manner. BE REASSURING AND SUPPORTIVE. If hyperventilating, then teach "brown paper lunch bag" rebreathing technique. Discuss stress reduction. Begin relaxation training. Provide educational materials. Synthesize a multifaceted approach/plan.

Specific Measures.
Give an Rx for _____*(MIS)
                                          or
_____*(MIS).

Physician Consultation. Severe agitation or severely symptomatic.

Referral. To therapist _____ for chronic recurring anxiety
                                          or
To psychiatrist _____ if dangerous to self or others, history of drug abuse

Immediate Transfer.

Follow-up Plan. Recheck in _____ days, sooner if worse.

                                                    Initials   Date
* unless allergic, contraindicated,   Physician
or pregnant/lactating   ARNP

Panic Attacks

EVALUATION/DIAGNOSTIC PROTOCOL
<u>Subjective</u>
History. Situational history (Why is the patient here now? and What does patient think is wrong?). Current medical history, past medical history, family history, family systems diagram and social history, psychiatric history (explore for presence of phobias (often multiple), avoidant behaviors and anticipatory anxiety), review of systems (dizziness, difficulty breathing, choking, chest discomfort/pain, palpitations, tachycardia, trembling, paresthesias, nausea, diaphoresis). Current medications: over the counter, prescription and illicit. Other substance use caffeine, alcohol and tobacco history.

<u>Objective</u>
Physical Examination. General appearance, vital signs (often elevated), neurologic exam (brisk reflexes), mental status exam (observing behavior, motor activity and affect including range and depth, thought content for obsessions, phobias, compulsive rituals and suicidal ideations) and symptom-specific system exam when complete physical exam is not possible.

Lab. Consider MMPI and full metabolic evaluation: CBC, chemistry panel, thyroid panel.

Assess presence, degree and sources of exogenous stimuli, severity and frequency of panic attacks (including degree of dysfunction and avoidant behavior), for phobia(s) type and severity. Does this meet DSM III-R criteria? Assess severity of psycho social stressors. Assess general functioning. **Differential Diagnosis**. Drug induced anxiety (caffeine, alcohol, nicotine, amphetamines, sympathomimetic agents, neuroleptic anitemetic agents, monosodium glutamate, and withdrawal phenomena), medical (hyperthyroidism, hypoglycemia, pheochromocytoma), psychiatric (agitated depression, hypomania, personality disorders, and psychoses). **Complications** include not only worsening dysfunction for the patient but also that for the family.

PLAN/MANAGEMENT PROTOCOL
General Measures. Conduct the history and physical examination in a non-judgmental manner. BE REASSURING AND SUPPORTIVE. Discuss panic disorders as a common psychiatric illness that is very responsive to treatment. Discuss the multifaceted therapeutic plan; educational readings, counseling and pharmacologic intervention.

Specific Measures
Consider an Rx for oral _____ *(MIS)
                                     coupled with/or
an Rx for _____ *(MIS) or alternative Rx _____ *(MIS).

Physician Consultation. For severe panic or severe dysfunction. For controlled substance prescriptions.

Referral. To therapist _____ or _____. Or to psychiatrist if symptomotology or severity warrant.

Immediate Transfer. If dangerous to self or others or if inpatient therapy indicated.

Follow-up Plan. Initially every _____ week(s) until therapeutic efficacy established and then every _____ month(s).

                                                    Initials   Date

* unless allergic, contraindicated,   Physician
or pregnant/lactating   ARNP

Depression

EVALUATION/DIAGNOSTIC PROTOCOL

Subjective

History. Situational psychiatric and situational social (Why is the patient here now? and What does the patient think is wrong?). Current medical history, past medical history, family history (of depression documented diagnosis or suspected), family system diagram and social and psychiatric history. The use of current medications, prescription and non-prescription, over the counter, or illicit. Review sleep habits (classically these are disturbed with difficulty falling asleep and staying asleep or excessive sleep). Review other symptoms (classically these include tiredness, irritability, sadness, difficulty concentrating, diminished sexual desire, and a number of different aches and pains). Any weight loss?

Objective

Physical Examination. General appearance, vital signs, neurologic exam, mental status exam (observe behavior, appearance, motoractivity, affect, thought content for hallucinations, delusions, suicidal or homocidal ideations with or without intent), "symptom specific" system exam when complete physical exam is not possible because of time limitation.

Lab. Usually none, but consider broad screening battery including CBC, chemistry panel, thyroid function tests (specifically).

Assessment. Try to assess the severity of depression, including degree of dysfunction and suicidal risk. Does this meet DSM III-R criteria? **Differential diagnosis** includes anemia, hypothyroidism, alcoholism, other substance abuse, and major psychosis. **Complications** include not only the dysfunction of the patient but emotional trauma to the family. The worst is suicide.

PLAN/MANAGEMENT PROTOCOL

General Measures. Conduct a history and physical examination in a non-judgmental manner. BE REASSURING AND SUPPORTIVE. Discuss depression as a common problem amongst adults which responds to a combination of pharmacotherapy and psychotherapy.

Specific Measures.
Consider Rx for oral antidepressant _____*(MIS)
                                              or
alternative antidepressant _____ or _____*(MIS).

Physician Consultation. For moderate to severe depression where patient severely symptomatic or suicidal.

Referral. To therapist _____ for counseling (if brief in-office psychotherapy not available) or if dangerous to self or others, history of drug or alcohol abuse, then refer to psychiatrist _____.

Immediate Transfer.

Follow-up Plan. Every _____ week(s) initially and then every _____ weeks or mos and prn.

                                                              Initials   Date

* unless allergic, contraindicated,   Physician
or pregnant/lactating   ARNP

Alcohol Abuse

EVALUATION/DIAGNOSTIC PROTOCOL
Subjective
History. Evaluation of abuse is facilitated by using one of many standard assessment questionnaires. At the least, find out if patient has thought about his or her drinking as a problem, been annoyed by others complaining about his or her drinking, felt guilty about drinking, or takes a drink before noon. If suspicion is present, obtain complete drinking history. Family alcohol history, drug history, signs and symptoms including physical, emotional, and mental.

Objective
Physical Examination. Vital signs and P/E as indicated to detect complications in stages of disease progression.

Lab. CBC with indices, chemistry panel, stool guiac tests. Consider serum amylase. Consider other drug screens.

Assess stage of disease versus potential for development of alcoholism; underlying factors related to patient's problem with alcohol use; readiness to accept diagnosis of alcoholism. **Differential Diagnosis**. **Complications** include malnutrition, hypoglycemia, gastrointestinal diseases, liver disease, pancreatitis, anemias, cardiovascular disease, hemorrhage, and fetal alcohol syndrome.

PLAN/MANAGEMENT PROTOCOL
General Measures. Confront the patient with the diagnosis of alcoholism or warn patient about potential for development of alcohol abuse. Devise treatment plan best suited to individual, utilizing support group such as AA, professional counseling, family involvement, and behavioral treatment approaches.

Specific Measures. For appropriate patients with physician consultation, consider Rx _____*(MIS).

Physician Consultation. Mid to late stage alcoholism or if complications are suspected.

Referral. Pending physician consultation, consider for inpatient detoxification program. Refer to mental health professional as indicated.

Immediate Transfer. Usually not necessary.

Follow-up Plan. Until evaluation of problem is complete and/or patient accepts diagnosis, every _____. If patient is not attending AA meetings or getting regular counseling every _____, otherwise follow up every _____.

	Initials	Date
* unless allergic, contraindicated, or pregnant/lactating	Physician ARNP	

Tobacco Abuse/Addiction

EVALUATION/DIAGNOSTIC PROTOCOL
Subjective
History. Smoking history, family history, past medical history including drug history, signs or symptoms indicative of possible complications.

Objective
Physical Examination. Vital signs and P/E as indicated by age and presentation.

Lab. As indicated--over 35, consider lipid profile, _____ and/or _____.

Assess patient's motivation level to quit, environmental support, individual risk factors. **Differential Diagnosis.** **Complications** include cardiovascular disease, lung disease, an increased risk for most types of cancer, exposure of others in close proximity to patient of toxic smoke.

PLAN/MANAGEMENT PROTOCOL
General Measures. Reinforce importance of quitting smoking during office visits--optimally at regular health maintenance exams. Realize that motivation of individual to quit is a necessity for success. Enlist family members in support of plan to maximize success. Detail physiologic damage done in plain terms without imposing moral tone. Forewarn most that they will gain some weight but less than 15% gain more than 10 kilos and that this can be modified with a successful exercise program and prudent diet. Frequent follow-up visits or enrollment in community program aimed at education and group support is advised. Devise with patient a list of alternative behaviors and explain usefulness of behavioral modification approach.

Specific Measures.
Consider Rx for _____*(MIS)
                                          or

consider a combined series of Rx's to modify anxiety and reduce withdrawal symptoms.

Physician Consultation. Not usually necessary.

Referral. To local "Stop Smoking" workshops or programs and as indicated for complications related to tobacco abuse.

Immediate Transfer. None.

Follow-up Plan. Initially every _____ weeks, then every _____ months or PRN.

	Initials	Date
* unless allergic, contraindicated,	Physician	
or pregnant/lactating	ARNP	

CHAPTER 15
OTHER INFECTIOUS AND PARASITIC DISEASES

Mumps

EVALUATION/DIAGNOSTIC PROTOCOL

Subjective

History. History of exposure (incubation period 2-3 weeks). Ascertain whether there are prodromal symptoms (fever, headaches, and weakness). Usually the main complaint relates to salivary gland involvement. Immunization history.

Objective

Physical Examination. General appearance, vital signs, ENT exam (with particular attention to salivary glands and ducts), abdominal exam and testicular exam.

Lab. Consider serologic testing for confirmation.

Assess severity. **Differential diagnosis** includes other disorders affecting the salivary glands. **Complications.** Orchitis, oophoritis, deafness, facial neuritis, myelitis, meningoencephalitis and pancreatitis.

PLAN/MANAGEMENT PROTOCOL

General Measures. Explain to patient and/or parents that mumps is a viral illness, generally benign although it may last as long as 14 days. Because it is easily spread the patient should be isolated for about a week after salivary swelling has subsided. It has been communicable 2-7 days prior to swelling. Report case to the local health department.

Encourage regular diet, but if chewing is too painful do not force eating. The acid tartness of citrus juices often hurts the salivary glands, so give other types of nourishing fluids, such as milk, milkshakes, cream soups.

Give acetaminophen in appropriate doses for age and weight.

Specific Measures. There is no specific therapy.

Physician Consultation. For patients with severe discomfort and those where diagnosis remains in doubt. Also obtain for patients with complications.

Referral.

Immediate Transfer. Usually not necessary.

Follow-up Plan. Follow-up is usually not necessary. Those developing complications should be seen immediately.

	Initials	Date
* unless allergic, contraindicated, or pregnant/lactating	Physician	
	ARNP	

Rubeola
Red Measles or Ten Day Measles

EVALUATION/DIAGNOSTIC PROTOCOL

Subjective

History. History of exposure (1-1/2 to 2 weeks). Ascertain whether there are prodromal symptoms (rising fever, rhinitis, cough, and conjunctivitis). The sicker patient will have anorexia, severe coughing, and lymphadenopathy. The rash begins on the face and neck, and spreads downward over the entire body. Only as the rash begins to fade does the patient begin to improve. Immunization history.

Objective

Physical Examination. General appearance (**usually very sick**), vital signs, eyes (conjunctival injection), ENT (during the prodrome Koplik's spots on the buccal mucosa, subsequently marked pharyngeal injection), neck, chest, abdomen, skin (macular papular dermatitis as discussed above begins on about the fourth day) that can become slightly hemorrhagic or petechial.

Lab. Consider acute and convalescent rubeola titers.

Assess severity. **Differential Diagnosis** is an attempt to distinguish this from the other viral exanthems. Note that the unimmunized may be very sick while those with partial immunity are less sick. Variant strains (wild) do occur and the accompanying symptoms ands signs are variable though usually milder. **Complications** include otitis media, corneal ulcers, obstuctive laryngitis, pneumonia, appendicitis, encephalomyelitis.

PLAN/MANAGEMENT PROTOCOL

General Measures. Explain to the patient and/or parents that measles is a viral illness, highly contagious (for the 3-5 days prior to rash and for 7-9 days after) , and usually making the patient quite ill.

Notify all contacts beginning with those when the patient had first signs of the prodome. This illness should be reported to your local health department even if you are not absolutely certain of the diagnosis so that the community can be protected.

Encourage a well-balanced diet and plenty of fluids. To make the patient more comfortable, treat fever with acetaminophen in appropriate dosages for age and weight). If the patient has light sensitivity, keep the room dark and limit close eye activity.

Specific Measures. There is no specific therapy.

Physician Consultation. On all suspected cases and again for all major complications.

Referral.

Immediate Transfer.

Follow-up Plan. Consider very close follow-up (to maintain isolation consider home visits or parking lot visits--go out to the car and auscultate their chests) and to monitor for signs of complications.

	Initials	Date
* unless allergic, contraindicated,	Physician	
or pregnant/lactating	ARNP	

Rubella
German Measles

EVALUATION/DIAGNOSTIC PROTOCOL

Subjective

History. History of exposure (incubation period 2-3 weeks). Ascertain any prodromal symptoms (usually none or slight fatigue, myalgias, coryza, but most characteristically there is lymphadenopathy in the retroauricular, posterior cervical or occipital areas), then fever and rash begin. The fever is usually mild, the rash is variable macula papular lesions beginning on the face but spreading quickly during the first day to cover the whole body. It clears in 3-5 days. Immunization history.

Objective

Physical Examination. General appearance, vital signs, ENT exam, neck exam with attention to lymphadenopathy in the previously mentioned areas, chest, abdomen, skin (for the rash described above).

Lab. Acute and convalescent rubella titers.

Assessment is directed at being certain of the diagnosis, **differentiating** this illness from the other viral exanthems and scarlet fever. **Complications** are rare for the patient with this illness. Though a transient polyarthritis is not uncommon However, complications are **very serious for pregnant women** in the first and second trimester.

PLAN/MANAGEMENT PROTOCOL

General Measures. Explain to the patient and/or parents that rubella is a viral illness that is generally benign. It is easily spread and the patient should be isolated until 5-7 days after the onset of the rash. Emphasize in absolute terms that all contacts must be notified, and in particular all adult women of child-bearing age, whether or not it is known if they are pregnant. Report illness to the local health department.

Encourage a well-balanced diet and plenty of fluids. The patient may have acetaminophen in appropriate dosages for weight or age.

Specific Measures. None.

Physician Consultation. For all suspected cases.

Referral.

Immediate Transfer.

Follow-up Plan.

	Initials	Date
* unless allergic, contraindicated, or pregnant/lactating	Physician	
	ARNP	

Roseola
Exanthum Subitum

EVALUATION/DIAGNOSTIC PROTOCOL
Subjective
History. The sequence of symptoms is critical to obtain. Classically, sudden onset of a very high fever (103-105 F/39.4-40.5 C) that lasts for several days. Usually there are no specific signs of the illness until the development of a maculopapular erythematous rash beginning on the trunk as the fever falls after about the third day. The rash then spreads somewhat. (Roseola is common amongst children between 6 months and 3 years of age.)

Objective
Physical Examination. General apperance, vital signs, eyes, ENT, neck, chest, abdomen, genitalia, skin (described above).

Lab. None necessary if definitive history of exposure. Otherwise the presentation of a very febrile child may be confusing and require considerable evaluation. (Consult attending.)

Assessment is difficult during the febrile phase. **Differential Diagnosis**. Literally includes all childhood illnesses. **Complications**. Febrile convulsions are not uncommon. Encephalitis is very rare.

PLAN/MANAGEMENT PROTOCOL
General Measures. Remind parents that as with all viruses there are no medications that affect roseola, and that the child should be isolated until the fever and rash have disappeared. Supportive measures, such as a well-balanced diet and plenty of fluids, will be helpful. Remind parents that at this level of fever extra fluids will be necessary. Give acetaminophen in appropriate dose for weight and age. Discuss other measures for reducing temperature, including lukewarm tub baths and dressing the child lightly.

Specific Measures. There are no specific measures.

Physician Consultation. Usually, as discussed above.

Referral.

Immediate Transfer.

Follow-up Plan. At the least, by phone daily until resolved.

	Initials	Date
* unless allergic, contraindicated, or pregnant/lactating	Physician ARNP	

Erythema Infectiosum
Fifth's Disease

EVALUATION/DIAGNOSTIC PROTOCOL

Subjective

History. The sequence of onset of symptoms and signs help establish this diagnosis. The patient may have a slight fever. The rash begins on the cheeks, giving them the look of having been slapped. Then it appears over the remainder of the body. It may last as long as three weeks, during which it will vary form a red flush to a lacy pink to being almost absent. The appearance of the rash can become worse after a hot bath, vigorous rubbing, if the child is upset or excited or exposed to bright sunlight. Some may have mild arthralgias.

Objective

Physical Examination. General appearance, vital signs, eyes, ENT, neck, chest, abdomen, genitalia, skin (described above).

Lab. None.

Assessment. This is a clinical diagnosis. **Differential Diagnosis.** Other exanthems and drug eruption. **Complications.** None for the child. This virus may affect pregnant woman and has been associated with first and second trimester miscarriages.

PLAN/MANAGEMENT PROTOCOL

General Measures. Explain that this is a benign viral illness. The fever is at the worst very mild and requires no treatment.

Notify contacts particularly woman of child-bearing age. Those trying to conceive should avoid contact for upwards of 10 days.

Specific Measures. There is no specific therapy.

Physician Consultation. Only if diagnosis remains unclear.

Referral.

Immediate Transfer.

Follow-up Plan. Usually not necessary.

Varicella
Chicken Pox

EVALUATION/DIAGNOSTIC PROTOCOL
Subjective
History. History of exposure (incubation period, 1-1/2 to 3 weeks). Ascertain whether there are/were prodromal symptoms (fever, lethargy, weakness, and anorexia). Usually the rash begins as individual red papules with subsequent tiny central vesicles. Determine how often the patient is having crops and which crop this is. Usually lesions occur first on the trunk, then spread to the face, scalp, extremities. They may involve mucus membranes.

Objective
Physical Examination. General appearance, vital signs, eyes, ENT, neck, chest, abdomen, genitalia, skin (pocks are as described above).

Lab. Usually none necessary.

Assess severity. **Differential Diagnosis** includes other vesicular eruptions when minimal. This disease can be confused with insect bites, herpes simplex, impetigo, when more generalized must be differentiated from other vesicular exanthems (Coxsackie, ECHO), erythema multiforme. **Complications** include very often secondary bacterial infection of the skin lesions. Pneumonia is a more common complication in adults. Rarer complications include Reye's syndrome and encephalitis.

PLAN/MANAGEMENT PROTOCOL
General Measures. Explain to the patient and/or parents that chicken pox is a viral illness. It is very easily spread and the patient should be isolated. The patient is contagious from onset of the prodrome until the pocks have stopped appearing and have crusted. Immune compromised contacts are at great risk and must be notified.

Patients may benefit from acetaminophen for fever and discomfort in appropriate dosage for weight and age. Caution against the use of aspirin.

A well-balanced diet should be encouraged. Parents should be cautioned if there are oral mucosal lesions that child may not eat well and plenty of neutral and nutritious fluids should be encouraged.

Remaining therapy is directed at the severe itching. Cornstarch or colloidal oatmeal baths may be helpful. Calamine lotion similarly may be helpful. The child's nails should be trimmed, and they should be discouraged from picking at the lesions.

Specific Measures.
Consider prescribing a mild antihistamine _____ *(MIS).
If secondary infection of skin lesions, consider prescribing _____ *(MIS).

Physician Consultation. For patients who seem severely ill or have complications other than secondary skin infection.

Referral.

Immediate Transfer.

Follow-up Plan. Necessary only if signs of secondary infections or Reye's syndrome (these include persistent vomiting, lethargy or incoherence).

	Initials	Date
* unless allergic, contraindicated, or pregnant/lactating	Physician ARNP	

Herpes Zoster

EVALUATION/DIAGNOSTIC PROTOCOL

Subjective

History. Determine the onset of sequence of symptoms. Itching or paresthesia (children often have minimal complaints; adults are more apt to have significant pain) in the dermatomal distribution of the rash can precede appearance of lesions by 3-5 days. Are there underlying or predisposing conditions? Review all medications, both prescription and nonprescription, that the patient has been using.

Objective

Physical Examination. General appearance, vital signs, and complete kin exam. In children it's preferable to perform a complete examination. Classically, the eruption covers a dermatomal pattern with the lesions beginning as red macules and progressing to papules with vesicles that often become papular.

Lab. When available, Tzanck prep is helpful, or consider biopsy or varicella zoster titers, acute and convalescent.

Assess severity. **Differential Diagnosis** includes herpes simplex and impetigo. **Complications** include life-threatening disseminated zoster. However, most complications relate to the location of the eruption and concomitant neuralgia. Postherpetic neuralgia is uncommon in children and most common in adults over 50.

PLAN/MANAGEMENT PROTOCOL

General Measures. Explain the usual course of zoster. Discuss compressing with Burrow's solution. Recommend acetaminophen in appropriate dosage for age or weight in children and adults. Explain the necessity to isolate the patient from potentially immune-compromised individuals.

Specific Measures.
When started early, oral Acyclovir _____*(MIS).

Consider an oral corticosteroid _____*(MIS)
(which may diminish risk for postherpetic neuralgia).

Physician Consultation. For children under 10, adults with cranial nerve involvement, any patient with severe pain or with underlying/predisposing conditions. Similarly, consult for management of postherpetic neuralgia.

Referral.

Immediate Transfer.

Follow-up Plan. Recheck every _____ days/weeks until considerable improved.

		Initials	Date
* unless allergic, contraindicated,	Physician		
or pregnant/lactating	ARNP		

Infectious Mononucleosis

EVALUATION/DIAGNOSTIC PROTOCOL

Subjective

History. Recent history of exposure to others with mononucleosis. Symptomatically patients usually focus on sore throat, swollen lymph nodes, and malaise. The incubation period is variable with reports varying from 5-15-30-45 days.

Objective

Physical Examination. General appearance, vital signs, ENT exam (exudative pharyngitis/tonsillitis), lymphoreticular exam (with particular attention to cervical lymph nodes and presence of hepatomegaly and especially splenomegaly), complete skin exam (variable maculopapular erythematous rash)

Lab. Complete blood count and some mono test _____ many mono test test for antibody that may take 3-5 days to develop. Also strep culture/test (25% of mono patients will also have positive strep).

Assess severity in the particular presence and degree of splenomegaly. **Differential Diagnosis** includes other prolonged viral syndromes, including hepatitis. **Complications.** Potential for spleenic rupture is the most life threatening. Others are aseptic meningitis and other neurologic sequale, hepatic and hematologic aberations, chronic EBV syndrome.

PLAN/MANAGEMENT PROTOCOL

General Measures. Explain the disease to patient and/or parent, emphasizing recovery comes with good nutrition and plenty of rest. Discuss a realistic schedule for rest and modifying school and/or work responsibilities.

It is of extreme importance to emphasize avoiding contact sports and other situations that could result in spleenic rupture, and minimize exertion.

Acetaminophen in appropriate dose for age and/or weight.

Specific Measures. Consider in the significantly ill child or those with marked tonsil hypertrophy and splenomegaly a short course of oral corticosteroid _____ _____*(MIS) with consult only.

Physician Consultation. Consult attending for toxic appearing or individual or marked splenomegaly. Consult if the diagnosis is unclear.

Referral

Immediate Transfer. Usually not necessary.

Follow-up Plan. Every _____ week(s) until considerably improved and in particular until splenomegaly resolved.

	Initials	Date
* unless allergic, contraindicated, or pregnant/lactating	Physician ARNP	

Enterobius vermicularis
(Pinworms)

EVALUATION/DIAGNOSTIC PROTOCOL
<u>Subjective</u>
History. Onset and course of symptoms (classically, nocturnal pruritis ani but may also present as restless sleep, nocturnal enuresis, vaginitis, diarrhea, vague abdominal pain, lower urinary tract symptoms, even masturbatory behavior).

<u>Objective</u>
Physical Examination. Exam as indicated.

Lab. Stool for parasites or microscopic evaluation of cellophane tape obtained by parents (as discussed below).

<u>Assess</u> severity. **Differential Diagnosis**. Monillia, anal fissure, dietary, infectious, or hygienic cause of perianal irritation. **Complications**. Perianal excoriations, secondary bacterial infections, vulvovaginitis.

PLAN/MANAGEMENT PROTOCOL
General Measures. Review with patient or parents that this is a nuisance problem, and usually without any significant sequelae. Review mechanism of transmission, specifically human to human by eggs which the female worm lays on the perianal skin when she crawls out of the rectum at night. These eggs get to the mouth by fingers that touch this area and then are swallowed by another human. Mostly this type of transfer occurs among young children. Swallowed eggs develop into adult worms in 2-4 weeks.

Parents can re-examine the child at night by shining a flashlight on the rectal area after the child has been asleep about an hour. The worms will be seen as tiny thread-like white worms 2 to 12 mm in length. An alternative is to press the sticky surface of cellophane tape against the rectum and the surrounding skin several times. The best time to use the tape is first thing in the morning.

On the day that treatment is prescribed, the family's night clothes and bed linens should be washed. Everyone should bathe thoroughly and trim their finger-nails.

Specific Measures
Consider treatment with an Rx _____*(MIS).
Also consider treating other family members.

Physician Consultation. Consider for recurrences or children intolerant of therapy.

Referral. Usually not necessary

Follow-up Plan. Parents should be instructed to call the doctor if they suspect the child has again developed pinworms. Reassure them this won't be an emergency and the office can be called during regular hours.

	Initials	Date
* unless allergic, contraindicated,	Physician	
or pregnant/lactating	ARNP	

Positive TB Screening Test
& Primary Pulmonary Tuberculosis

EVALUATION/DIAGNOSTIC PROTOCOL
Subjective
History. History of known exposure (incubation may be as long as several months). Are there any predisposing factors (chronic respiratory disease, chronic inhalant exposure, immunologically impaired particularly HIV infection)? Particular detail should be given to the respiratory and constitutional symptomotology though most primary infections are nearly asymptomatic. Obtain Tb test history and if has lived abroad whether BCG had been previously administered.

Objective
Physical Examination. Complete with particular attention to chest specifically and the lymphoreticular system.

Lab. Urinalysis, chest x-ray (track previous films for comparison) (for detection of the common forms of pediatric in thoracic TB including the most common localized noncalcified focus which in infants and young children often is peripheral and in adolescents apical or infraclavicular either with accompanying intrathoracic adenopathy) and subsequently consider intradermal PPD. Consider HIV test.

Assessment is directed at the accuracy of the screening test but more importantly at whether the patient has resolving or resolved primary tuberculosis or is indolent or progressive. **Differential Diagnosis** is based on the reaction to the intradermal test: 10 mm or >10 is positive for M. tuberculosis, 5 mm to 9 mm is doubtful, 0 mm to 4 mm usually negative. Repeat in _____ months (beware anergic response). These criteria are different in the immune-compromised. (An anergy control battery should be placed, too.) Note that Tb can occur in many forms. This DDx is for pulmonary forms and is still very broad but includes infections (viral, bacterial, fungal, protozoal), malignancy, foreign material, aspiration, scarring. **Complications** are an adverse reaction to the intradermal test or those as a result of inaccurate testing and false negative results pleuritis, infiltrative pneumonia, cavitary abscess, generalized spread (miliary) and death.

PLAN/MANAGEMENT PROTOCOL
General Measures involve educating the patient and or parents and significant others about the significance of the positive test result and or the primary infection. Also, educate about the importance of following through the recommended treatments and subsequent appointments. Dispel myths and above all be positive this no longer "consumption." Address special circumstances such as pregnancy. Note a very different discussion is required for the immune compromised and the HIV infected patient.

Specific Measures. Isoniazid for Tb test converters (and close contacts of active cases) under age 35 or regardless of age in those newly infected, or with past history but not treated (or chest x-ray evidence of same), or those at increased risk. Length of course varies with circumstance and dose varies with age and weight. There are absolute contraindications to isoniazid. Multiple drug therapy is employed in other circumstances (consult standard references and public health authorities or current CDC guidelines).

Physician Consultation. The authors recommend considering for all cases unless detailed diagnostic and therapeutic guidelines have been established for your practice setting.

Referral.

Follow-up Plan. Determined by the patient's underlying conditions and specific therapy prescribed.

	Initials	Date
* unless allergic, contraindicated, or pregnant/lactating	Physician ARNP	

HIV Positive

The authors find it particularly difficult to construct a detailed protocol on this problem to be confined to a single page; nevertheless the burgeoning presence of this disease requires that every primary care provider evolve an approach.

EVALUATION/DIAGNOSTIC PROTOCOL

Subjective

History. Complete medical history to include general history, past medical history (surgeries, hospitalizations and or transfusions), social history with detailed sexual history and substance use history, occupational exposure. Review of systems including a psychiatric history. Immunization history.

Objective

Physical Examination. General appearance, eye, ENT (oral lesions), lymphoreticular, Pulmonary, cardiovascular, abdominal, genitourinary, anorectal, dermatologic, neurologic, mental status.

Lab. Should have included a western blot which was positive. Tests to establish baseline parameters including CD4, CBC with differential, chemistry panel, urinalysis, RPR or VDRL, hepatitis screening, toxoplasmosis titers. Also chest x-ray and IPPD with anergy controls.

Assessment. The stage according to CDC: Stage I indicates acute infection, Stage II indicates asymptomatic infx, and Stage III indicates persistent generalized lymphadenopathy any of these can follow an early care protocol. **Differential Diagnosis** depends on the stage of infection and/or the ARC or AIDS-related condition(s) or specific defining conditions in those patients beyond Stage III. **Complications** include many opportunistic infections (e.g., pneumocystis carinii pneumonia [PCP], tuberculosis, atypical mycobacteria) and associated malignancies and the other ARC or AIDS-defining conditions.

PLAN/MANAGEMENT PROTOCOL

General Measures. Try to encourage the patient to lead a normal lifestyle with plenty of rest and good nutrition and plenty of exercise. In particular, counsel about those behaviors which put others at risk.

Address the psychosocial and psychiatric stress of this illness. Recommend counseling. Emphasize those issues that they can control, such as compliance with the recommendations made for regular monitoring and medications.

Provide access to reliable patient resource materials (e.g., CDC AIDS Information Line, 1-800-342-AIDS).

Specific Measures

Consider zidovudine (per CDC guidelines) _____ *(MIS).
Note that AIDS Clinical Trials Information Service (ACTIS) can provide additional information (1-800-TRIALS-A).

Follow appropriate CDC/NIAID immunologic prophylaxis guidelines.

Physician Consultation on all newly diagnosed patients. And certainly for those with ARC of AIDS.

Referral.

Immediate Transfer.

Follow-up Plan. Will be determined by patient's personal needs, staging, and specific therapy instituted.

	Initials	Date
* unless allergic, contraindicated, or pregnant/lactating	Physician ARNP	

Lyme Disease

EVALUATION/DIAGNOSTIC PROTOCOL
<u>Subjective</u>
History. Was there a tick bite? Is it an endemic area for Lyme disease? When did it occur? What symptoms have been noted (specifically, flu-like symptoms or expanding skin lesion, early stage; cardiac and neurological symptoms, second stage; arthritis and chronic neurological symptoms, third stage)? General medical history. Medications, prescription and otherwise. Family history.

<u>Objective</u>
Physical Examination. Vital signs, general appearance. Skin, muscular-skeletal, cardiovasvular, and neuro exam.

Lab. Usually Borrelia burgdorferi serologic tests (may not be positive in early stages of disease and the reliability of these tests is currently in question--THIS DIAGNOSIS IS OFTEN A CLINICAL ONE). Consider CBC, chemistry panel, ANA, RA latex, Sed rate, uric acid.

<u>Assessment</u>. What is the likelihood that the tick bite has infected the patient with Borrelia burgdorferi producing Lyme disease? Stage of disease. **Differential Diagnosis.** Influenza, infected tick bite not caused by Ixodid tick, other arthritic, cardiac, or neurological problems. **Complications.** Progression to second or third stage; antibiotic therapy most effective in early stages.

PLAN/MANAGEMENT PROTOCOL
General Measures. Discuss cause and treatment of disease. Educate patients and their families about prevention, especially if you are in an endemic area (protective, light-colored clothing, tick repellent, careful checking when undressing). If treating cardiac, neurological, or arthritic manifestations, facilitate referrals, review disease process with patient/family, and stress importance of taking medications.

Specific Measures. TREAT WITH ANTIBIOTICS IF THERE IS REASONABLE CLINICAL SUSPICION THAT THE PATIENT HAS EARLY LYME DISEASE.
Nonpregnant, nonlactating women and children over eight _____*(MIS).
Children, pregnant, and lactating women _____*(MIS).

If allergic to tetracyclines or penicillins _____*(MIS).
For later stages _____*(MIS).

Physician Consultation. For diagnostic uncertainty; if there are signs of late stage disease; if not responding to treatment.

Referral. Consider to _____.

Immediate Transfer.

Follow-up Plan. Every _____ days until symptoms are resolved or as indicated by condition.

		Initials	Date
* unless allergic, contraindicated, or pregnant/lactating	Physician ARNP		

CHAPTER 16
PATIENT INSTRUCTION SHEETS

Suture Care Sheet

Your/your child's cut (laceration) requires stitches (sutures) to promote more rapid healing. Though it will not prevent the formation of a scar, the result should be better than if the wound had been left open.

The location and nature of your/your child's injury may require that the wound be rechecked in a certain number of days. The stitches usually should be removed in a specific number of days. Ask about when to make these appointments.

Keep the wound dry. Leave the original dressing on as long as it appears clean. Otherwise, the dressing should be changed every _____ day(s).

You may take or may give your child acetaminophen--the common aspirin substitute--in appropriate doses for age or weight to help relieve discomfort.

Healing will cause the wound to itch. You should not or your child should not scratch or pick at it.

When to Call the Doctor Again
Though most wounds will ooze some tissue fluid, the practitioner or doctor should be contacted if there is pus.

Though it is natural to have discomfort with any wound, and particularly after the numbing injection wears off, continued pain is another reason for calling the doctor. Call also if the area around the wound swells, becomes red, or your child develops a fever.

Stitches should be rechecked in _____ day(s).

Stitches will be removed in _____ day(s).

From Instructions for Parents, Second Edition, to be published in July 1992, by permission of Sunbelt Medical Publishers, Tallahassee, Florida.

Minor Head Injury and Concussion Syndrome Instructions

The patient should be observed every _____ hour(s) for the next _____ hours. This includes awakening the patient. Similarly over subsequent _____ day(s), the patient should just be generally observed for the following:

1. Difficult to awaken by ordinary means
2. Vomiting more than once or twice after the first few hours
3. Headache unrelieved by acetaminophen
4. Pupil of one eye bigger than the other
5. Neck stiffness
6. Fever of 101 F° (38 C°) or greater
7. Convulsion
8. Dizziness that persists
9. Confusion or other personality change
10. Weakness in an arm or leg compared to that on the other side
11. Speech difficulty
12. Visual difficulty

Should any of these signs or symptoms develop, your doctor should be contacted immediately. Usually minor head trauma with concussion syndrome does not result in any permanent damage. The above signs or symptoms could mean the injury is more serious.

From Instructions for Parents, Second Edition, to be published in July 1992, by permission of Sunbelt Medical Publishers, Tallahassee, Florida.

YOUR NEWBORN

Each newborn is an individual. Your baby probably looks different from what you expected. At birth, its skin is covered with a thick, white, creamy substance called vernix, which, when removed, leaves a reddened, puffy, curled-up being -- your new baby.

Your baby's **body** may be covered with fine, downy hair (lanugo). The amount, color, and areas covered vary. The lanugo is shed naturally during the first weeks. The hands and feet may be bluish and cold because of immature circulation.

The **skin** may become dry and wrinkled because of the change from the moist womb environment to room air. It is not necessary to rub the skin and scalp with oil.

Approximately 40% of all babies may have a rash during the first few weeks consisting of small, raised, white spots on the face (milia). This is the normal beginning of the function of oil and sweat glands. No treatment is needed as these spots disappear on their own (and should not be squeezed).

Fifty percent of all babies may have a rash consisting of red, raised patches (erythema toxicum). This rash begins during the first days of life and usually disappears within a week. The rash frequently occurs on the chest, abdomen, back, or bottom. No treatment is needed.

Babies are born with different amounts of hair. Some babies are even bald. The scalp hair may be rubbed away, in patches, as your baby shifts its head about. The hair color at birth is often different from that in childhood. Newborn fingernails are thin and long from growth in the womb.

The **head** appears large in relation to your baby's body. Because of the head's weight, it needs support when the baby is handled. The head may be misshapen because passage through the birth canal has molded the soft bones. This is normal and the skull will round out during the next year. The brain has not been damaged. If your baby favors lying in a particular position, that side of the skull may appear flat. This, too, returns to normal as the bones mature. There are two soft spots (fontanelles) in the head where the brain is covered by a tough membrane until bone grows over them during the next year. The size of the soft spot is different for each child. There is no danger in washing or combing the skin and hair of these areas.

The color of the **eyes** at birth may be different from that as an adult. Most newborns have eyes that are gray-blue or, if they are darker complected, brown in color. Occasionally, there will be a red blood spot (hemorrhage) in the white of one eye. This is due to the breaking of a tiny blood vessel that often occurs during the birth process. Though the spot looks bad, it will resolve without treatment. Passage through the birth canal often causes considerable swelling of the eyelids which will take several days to resolve. Occasionally, swelling, mattering, or tearing from both eyes may be due to the eye drops used at birth. Coordination of your baby's eye movements develops gradually over the next year.

The newborn's **face** is usually rounded with the cheeks being pudgy. In the first few days, the lips will begin to form sucking callouses which look like tiny blisters. Occasionally, a baby's tongue is short but will lengthen with age. This rarely causes speech difficulties (contrary to popular misconception). Your baby's teeth will not break through the gums for many months.

In some babies, during the ensuing days, the **breasts** become enlarged and may secrete a milky substance. This is due to the transmission of the mother's hormones prior to delivery. Do not massage or squeeze the breasts.

The __umbilical cord__ was the connection from the baby to the placenta inside the uterus. Though glistening white at birth, it turns brown during the first few days as it dries. If kept dry, it will fall off during the first few weeks. Some people dab it with alcohol, using a cotton ball or swab, several times daily to aid this drying process. At the time the cord falls off, it is normal to see some blood-like drops on the raw naval, clothing, or diaper. Continue to keep the raw area dry and clean until it heals. If the area of attachment develops a bad odor, redness, or pus, contact your practitioner/physician. Do not tub bathe your infant until the raw area has healed. Many babies, particularly black infants, have an out-pouching of the belly button area (umbilical hernia). This hernia is due to a gap in the muscles of the abdominal wall around the naval. Most of these hernias disappear on their own during the first few years.

Often the __genitals__ will seem large in comparison to the rest of the body. Females may have a discharge from the vagina varying from white to red or brown in color. This is also due to the influence of the mother's hormones and usually starts and stops in the first few weeks.

In a male infant whose penis has been circumcised, the edge will take a number of days to heal. Care should be taken to prevent irritation of the wound. Wash and dry this area gently. A dab of antibiotic ointment or petroleum jelly on the wound will prevent it from sticking to the diaper. If not circumcised, it is not necessary to retract your child's foreskin. It is normal, and of no significance, for erections to occur.

The __arms__ and __legs__ will often temporarily stay in a position similar to that in the womb. The legs may be bowed for the same reason. The feet, too, may be at an odd angle. As your child matures, particularly after walking has begun, the feet and legs return to more normal positions.

Though your infant looks helpless and is dependent on you for most of his/her needs, there are a number of __things babies can do__. They possess language, communicating with you by crying various ways. Each cry is different in characteristic. There is one to get attention, to feed, or for just being uncomfortable. Babies may normally have fussy periods during each day when they cry for variable amounts of time without apparent reason. Most commonly, this occurs in the late afternoon or early evening when the household is least relaxed.

Your baby can perform the __basic life functions__ of breathing, sucking, swallowing, keeping warm, and expelling waste. These functions are performed with a pattern of regularity peculiar to your child. Your infant's normal breathing pattern will vary, just like yours. Your child has the ability to see, hear, taste, smell, and feel. Newborns are quite capable of movements. A number of these are involuntary reflexes: rooting (turning the head toward that cheek which is touched as a prelude to feeding), sucking, startling to sudden contact or noise (known as the Moro reflex), withdrawing the limbs (a means of protection), grasping, blinking, yawning, gagging, coughing, and sneezing. The degree of active movement varies with each individual. Hiccups is another normal process which stops on its own.

With all this activity as well as considerable growth, it is no surprise that the average newborn sleeps 12 to 18 hours a day.

The frequency and intensity of these behaviors is different because each newborn is an individual.

From __Instructions for Parents__, Second Edition, to be published in July 1992, by permission of Sunbelt Medical Publishers, Tallahassee, Florida.

Newborn Care

Caring for your newborn is a challenging job. When awake, your baby will need feeding, changing, cleaning, and variety of stimulation. It is through his/her senses that your baby learns about life. Give your infant the necessary time and plenty of loving.

Your Baby's Environment
Both you and your baby need time to yourselves. If an extra room is available, make it into a nursery. Try to make the nursery a place that will be exciting to your child with brightly colored objects, mobiles, and other stimuli.

Your baby's room should be kept at a comfortable temperature (68° to 72° F or 20° to 22° C). During the winter the heat at home is drying, so use a cool mist humidifier where your child sleeps. In the hot summer, the room should be well ventilated.

There is no need to confine the baby to the nursery. You can give your child varied experiences by providing new environments such as a play area and other rooms at home or at a friend's house. Also take your infant outside when the weather is nice. Special protection may be necessary when taking your infant out in cold weather (appropriate winter clothing) or in bright sunlight.

Sleeping
There is considerable confusion among parents and in print about infant sleep positions. Your baby probably has a preferred sleeping position in which he/she is most comfortable. It is not necessary to place your infant in another position unless so instructed by your practitioner or physician. It is best for infants to sleep on a firm mattress. A pillow should not be used because your infant may not be able to lift his/her head out of it.

If you go about your daily business as usual, your child will become accustomed to sleeping with household sounds. If you are tired or have no other children or responsibilities, use your baby's nap time to rest.

Cleanliness
Until your child's cord has come off and the navel heals, it is best to only sponge bathe the baby. Remember, a soapy baby is a slippery baby. It is a good idea to rest your child on a towel while sponging. It is not necessary to bathe your baby daily.

Real bathing can be done in any object that holds water and is convenient, such as a large pan, sink, or baby tub. Again, placing a towel or washcloth on the bottom of the tub will make it less slippery. When using a sink, be sure the how water spigot has cooled. ALWAYS TEST THE BATH WATER TO BE SURE THAT IT IS NOT TOO HOT! Use a mild soap and infant washcloth for bathing. For shampooing, the same soap or a mild shampoo will be find. Bath time should be a stimulating, cheerful, wet experience for both you and your child.

There is often considerable concern about caring for the ears. They should be cleansed by gently using a washcloth. It is not necessary to clean the canal with cotton swabs. Wax is a normal product of the ears and is not dirt. The nose, too, can be adequately cleansed using a washcloth. In general, it is not necessary to clean, prod, or dig mucus out of the nostrils. In girls, use the washcloth to clean the genitals, particularly between the lips (labia), washing from front to back.

After bathing, pat dry with a soft towel. It is not necessary to powder, lotion, or oil your baby. Some infants' skin is sensitive to these substances. Sometimes these provide a place for infections to begin. If you feel compelled to rub something on your child, use a lotion: a petroleum jelly or oil does not allow the skin to breathe. If you feel compelled to powder your baby, use cornstarch or cornstarch-based powder; the talc in some powders is harmful if inhaled.

At first, it will be necessary to cut the nails frequently. This is best done using blunt infant nail scissors or nail clippers when the baby is asleep or sleepy as there may be less of a struggle. Cut the nails in a straight line rather than curves, which contribute to ingrowing.

Clothing

Your baby needs to be dressed comfortably for the temperature that he/she is experiencing. Usually this means dress as you dress, in less clothing than you think the baby needs and much less clothing than grandparents thing he/she needs! A baby's hands and feet often feel cool. Feel his/her chest or back to see whether your baby is really cold.

Your infant's clothes should be washed only in mild detergent. It is a good idea to wash all new clothes before your child wears them. This removes any of a number of possible irritants.

Diaper

Because most newborns wet frequently, they may require diaper changing 15 to 20 or more times each day. The number and type of bowel movements will vary according to what your child is fed. Formula-fed infants move their bowels on the average of 1 to 4 times a day. Breast-fed babies will have a movement as often as every feeding, which will be light yellow and pasty in consistency, or infrequent movements every 2 to 5 days of the same consistency. It is common for bowels to move after feeding since this stimulates the intestinal tract. It is normal for your infant to appear to grunt and strain. As long as the movement is soft, he/she is not constipated.

It is important to clean the baby after each bowel movement. Use a washcloth, cotton balls, or tissue moistened with lukewarm water. Wipe gently from front to back. If your baby has sensitive skin, you may just need to bathe his/her bottom when changing a diaper.

Soiled diapers should be rinsed in the toilet before they are placed in the diaper pail. Diapers should be washed with mild soap or detergent. If they are washed by hand, rinse enough to get the water clear. If you are using a machine, wash with hot water. When bleaching, use a double rinse. Diapers can be line dried for sun bleaching; avoid chemicals. Many babies are sensitive to fabric softeners. Diaper services and disposable diapers are nice conveniences.

Feeding

Feeding is a subject that deserves further discussion and other educational materials should be made available to you.

Other Care

Other problems surrounding the care of your infant should be discussed with your practitioner/doctor. It is helpful for you to write down your questions and their answers. You may also benefit from consulting some other baby care references.

From <u>Instructions for Parents</u>, Second Edition, to be published in July 1992, by permission of Sunbelt Medical Publishers, Tallahassee, Florida.

Fever in Children

Fever is an elevation of your child's temperature beyond normal. Normal temperature is orally 98.6° F or 37° C and rectally 99.2° F or 37.3° C. A fever is seldom significant if it cannot be felt by the hand. But you cannot accurately tell the extent of fever by touch. Therefore check your child's temperature with a thermometer. Fever is a symptom of an illness, most commonly an infection. Fever in babies under six months of age can be an indication of a serious illness and your child's practitioner/doctor should be contacted promptly.

In part, the fever represents your child's immune defenses responding to illness. Consequently, a fever often needs reduction solely for your child's comfort. Fevers themselves usually are not harmful (they don't cause brain damage). Reducing the fever alone does not eliminate its cause. The cause of the fever must be determined and treated appropriately. However, it is important to keep the fever within reasonable limits, particularly if it exceeds 102° F or 38.8° C, which becomes quite uncomfortable for your child.

A number of simple measures may be taken to help control a fever. You should dress your child **lightly** to allow the body heat to escape. That's right! It is a misconception to bundle the child to cause the fever to burn out. Keep the room temperature cool. Encourage your child to drink plenty of fluids, particularly cool fluids such as favorite juices or sodas.

Bathing your child in lukewarm water is more comfortable to the child than sponging or rubbing with alcohol. (Alcohol fumes can be dangerous.) Immerse as much of the body, except the head, in the bath as possible. (Cold water enemas can be dangerous and should not be used.)

You should use acetaminophen--the common aspirin substitute (never use aspirin)--in doses appropriate for your child's weight or age. These should be used every four to six hours if the temperature rises about 102° F (38.8° C) orally, 102.6° F (39.2° C) rectally. These medicines and the above measures only help reduce a fever. Often these do not bring the temperature to normal. These measures do not prevent the temperature from rising again.

You should contact your practitioner/doctor if your child appears severely ill and/or has alarming symptoms other than fever. If the cause of your child's fever is apparent, such as a cold, it is not necessary to call. However, if your child's condition worsens at any time or does not improve within three days, the practitioner/doctor should be contacted. If the fever lasts more than 24 hours without apparent cause or if you are unable to reduce fever below 104° F (40.0° C) orally, 104.6° F (40.3 C) rectally, your practitioner/doctor should also be promptly contacted.

From Instructions for Parents, Second Edition, to be published in July 1992, by permission of Sunbelt Medical Publishers, Tallahassee, Florida.

Middle Ear Infection, Infants and Children
(Otitis Media)

What Is It?
Otitis media is an infection of the portion of the ear behind the drum--the middle ear. This infection often follows the common cold, sinus trouble, sore throats, and tonsillitis, all of which can extend to the middle ear via the tube connecting it to the back of the throat (eustachian tube). Inflammation and swelling of the eustachian tube itself causes changes in the pressure in the middle ear which strain the eardrum causing pain.

What Are the Symptoms?
Young children do not localize pain well and may just manifest a fever and/or be irritable. These children may awake frequently throughout the night. Occasionally there will be vomiting and diarrhea. Older children may complain of pain in the region of the ear, hearing loss (usually temporary), or just pull at the ears. Other ear diseases can cause similar symptoms.

How Long Does It Last?
Most acute otitis media respond rapidly to treatment, for the most part showing considerable improvement during the initial week, though the changes caused by the infection may take several weeks or months to clear.

What Are the Complications?
When adequately treated, middle ear infections rarely cause permanent damage. Sometimes fluid will continue to accumulate in the middle ear even after the infection has cleared because of eustachian tube malfunction. This fluid accumulation may require additional medical treatment and, occasionally, surgical drainage.

Occasionally, buildup of fluid behind the drum and pressure can cause rupture (perforation) of the eardrum (tympanic membrane). The eardrum usually heals quickly within the next few weeks without permanent damage or hearing loss. The healing process should be watched closely by the doctor.

Rarely do more serious complications occur.

How Common Is It?
Middle ear infections are quite common in infants and young children because of the immature anatomy of the eustachian tubes. Some children seem more prone to otitis media than others, particularly those infants who receive feedings with propped bottles, those children with nasal allergies, and those in homes with a smoker.

What Has the Doctor Done?
Some physicians use anesthetic drops to soothe the painful eardrum. Your practitioner/doctor will prescribe an antibiotic either by injection or by mouth, usually the latter. If by mouth, bring the bottle with you on the next visit.

What Can the Family Do?

Initial treatment usually includes a medicine to relieve the pain and control fever, such as aspirin or acetaminophen (the common aspirin substitute). Your child should be given the entire course of antibiotics prescribed. Many doctors use oral decongestants which help keep the eustachian tube open, relieving the pressure in the ear. Sometimes the older child can open the tube just by blowing his/her own nose. Another way is for the child to pinch the nostrils closed and then to try to gently blow air into the ears. Occasionally the eardrum must be opened surgically to drain pus.

When To Call the Doctor Again

Fever, pain, headache, and dizziness are common, but, if persistent, you should notify your practitioner/physician. Remember, the young child with persistent symptoms may have only irritability and/or frequent awakenings. Make an appointment to have your child rechecked in _____ days to see that the infection has resolved and that there are no continuing problems.

From Instructions for Parents, Second Edition, to be published in July 1992, by permission of Sunbelt Medical Publishers, Tallahassee, Florida.

Swimmer's Ear Infection
(Otitis Externa)

What Is It?
Otitis externa is an inflammation of the ear canal. This inflammation can be due to infection by a virus, bacteria, or fungus. Otitis externa may occur as a result of the loss of protective ear wax, injury to the skin of the canal, and subsequent infection. Immersion (swimmer's ear) often causes water to accumulate behind the wax or between the wax and the skin, creating moisture damage to the skin and providing a place for infection to begin. Injury can also occur from cotton swabs or other objects used to clean the ear. Infection of the ear canal can also spread from middle ear infections or from infections or rashes outside the ear.

What Are the Symptoms
The patient with otitis externa complains of pain or throbbing in the involved ear. Your child may also have fever, swollen glands (lymph nodes) below the ear, and headache around the ear. It is characteristic that an traction (tugging) on the ear will make the pain or pressure on the ear in front of the canal considerably worse. Some individuals have a chronic otitis externa, which may cause their ear to be uncomfortable, itch, and have a foul discharge.

How Long Does It Last?
Most ear canal infections respond rapidly to treatment, showing considerable improvement during the first week.

What Are the Complications?
Usually there are no serious complications.

How Common Is It?
Some people seem more prone than others to recurrences of otitis externa. Most people experience this type of problem at one time or another.

What Has the Doctor Done?
Your practitioner/doctor will need to remove some of the infected material or, if this is painful, may temporarily insert a medicated wick. The wick will help keep the medicine in contact with the infected walls of the canal. Eardrops containing antibiotics or other antiinfective and soothing agents are prescribed. Occasionally for severe infections, antibiotics will be prescribed to be taken by mouth.

What Can the Family Do?
Treatment includes a medicine to relieve the pain, such as acetaminophen (the common aspirin substitute), which will also help control the fever. The ears must be kept dry. This can be done by wearing a shower cap or bathing cap. After showering or swimming, the older child or adult may dry his/her ears by holding a hair dryer on the warm setting directed toward the canal, at the manufacturer's recommended distance.

Ear wax is a natural body substance that usually need not be removed. Cleaning can be performed on the outer ear using nothing smaller than a finger covered with a washcloth. Many doctors recommend that a few drops of a solution that is 1/2 rubbing alcohol and 1/2 white vinegar be put in each ear after swimming or showering. Be care not to get in the eyes. The alcohol helps to evaporate the water and the vinegar changes the acidity.

When To Call the Doctor Again
Call the doctor if pain continues despite the use of acetaminophen, or if the ear has a persistent discharge. Recheck in _____ days for wick removal or in _____ days if not considerably improved.

From _Instructions for Parents_, Second Edition, to be published in July 1992, by permission of Sunbelt Medical Publishers, Tallahassee, Florida.

The Common Cold, Children

What Is It?
The common cold is an infection of the nose and throat. Over 120 different viruses can cause colds. At present no medications are available that cure these colds.

What Are the Symptoms?
There are a number of symptoms caused by cold viruses, including a running or stuffed nose, sneezing, sore throat, cough, hoarseness, fever, feeling tired (lethargy), and loss of appetite.

How Long Does It Last?
Most colds are self-limiting. The average cold lasts 2 to 14 days but improvement is usually noted after the first few days.

What Are the Complications?
Cold viruses can lower resistance to infections from bacteria that can cause pneumonia and to infections of the bronchial tree, sinuses, or ears.

How Common Is It?
Some children seem more likely than others to get colds. The average child has 3 to 10 colds each year and as many as 100 by age 10. Colds are more common in the winter because of the increased exposure to others with colds that occurs indoors.

Children who live in a home where there are one or more smokers often have three times as many upper respiratory infections as other children. They inhale what the smoker does not and thus overload the respiratory system's ability to handle infections.

How Is It Acquired?
Colds are spread from one person to another. The viruses are transmitted by droplets sprayed in the air, from the nose with sneezes, or from the mouth with coughs. They can also be spread from nose or mouth by hand to another individual. Wash your hands frequently.

What Can the Family Do?
There is no specific therapy for colds. To protect others, keep your child home until symptoms subside and normal activities are resumed. Encourage large amounts of fluids, particularly favorite juices, soft drinks, gelatin desserts, popsicles, and soups. Extra fluids help replace the water lost with a fever. A well-balanced diet helps, but do not force eating; a lack of appetite is common with illness. Encourage your child to get rest and plenty of sleep. Quiet play, even outside the house, will not be harmful.

The fever should be treated with acetaminophen (the common aspirin substitute) in appropriate dosage for weight and age. Tepid baths also help absorb extra heat and are not as uncomfortable as sponging. In the winter, the indoor heat and fever may dry and irritate the nose and throat. Keep the room temperature between 68° and 70° F (20° to 21° C). Moistening the air in the bedroom will help. This is best accomplished with a cool-mist humidifier, which is inexpensive and considerably less dangerous than a hot vaporizer.

Young infants may need gentle suction with a rubber bulb aspirator to clear the nose, especially before eating or sleeping. This can be purchased at any drugstore. When using, squeeze the bulb before inserting into the nostril so that mucus will be sucked out, not pushed in. Most children gain little from the oral medicines that shrink the nasal passages and dry mucus but do not affect the cold virus. Additionally, these medicines may alter your child's behavior, making him/her irritable or sleepy. Medicines which suppress coughing are harmful (because the cough helps to clear breathing passages) and should only be used if the cough prevents your child from sleeping. Chest rubs have little or no value.

Many doctors recommend salt water (saline) nose drops for infants. These should be <u>made fresh daily</u> by adding 1/2 teaspoon of table sale to 8 ounces (240 milliliters) of water. Put 2 to 4 drops in each nostril just prior to feeding your infant and suck the drops and moistened mucus out with the rubber bulb aspirator four times each day.

Commercial nose drops or nasal sprays should never be used in infants or toddlers. In older children these drops and sprays often aggravate congestion if used for longer than three days. After three days, throw the drops or spray away.

When To Call the Doctor Again

If your child does not improve in the first few days, is becoming worse, acting more irritable, or looking more sickly, or if there is severe coughing, ear complaints, or persistent high fever above 102° F (38.8° C) then the physician needs to be consulted promptly.

From <u>Instructions for Parents</u>, Second Edition, to be published in July 1992, by permission of Sunbelt Medical Publishers, Tallahassee, Florida.

Allergy-Proofing the Bedroom

1. The bedroom must be completely empty of extra furniture, rugs, carpets, drapes, and curtains. Empty the closets and store as much as possible elsewhere or in tight containers.

2. Clean the walls, woodwork, and floors. Every inch must be spic and span. The floor should be wet-mopped and waxed.

3. The bed and the springs should be scrubbed. The mattress, unless it is made out of foam rubber, must be enclosed in a plastic air-proof cover. The box springs should be covered in plastic. The pillows should be hypo-allergenic, Dacron, polyester, or foam (definitely not feathers). Blankets should be synthetic fiber and not wool. Sheets should be cotton and/or polyester. Do not use chenille bedspreads. Do not use quilts or comforters unless the batting is synthetic.

Preferably the room should contain only one bed. If another bed is in the room, it should be prepared in the same way.

4. Keep the amount of furniture to a minimum. Do not use upholstered furniture, only wood or plastic, which are easily cleaned.

5. Use only washable throw rugs if a rug must be used. Drapes and curtains must be washable. Plastic shades or curtains are best. Venetian blinds should be removed permanently. Rugs and curtains must be washed weekly.

6. Thoroughly dust daily by damp-wiping and wash weekly the bedroom floors and walls. Do these things when your child is out of the room.

7. Keep windows and doors closed as much as possible.

8. Never allow pets in the bedroom.

9. Keep dust collectors out of the bedroom. This includes books and stuffed animals. The latter should be eliminated entirely. Washable toys are preferable.

10. Air conditioning with electrostatic filters is very helpful. Make sure that the heating system has effective filtering. An additional filter over the outlet to the bedroom is helpful. This can be made from several layers of cheese-cloth. Change or clean filters according to manufacturer's recommended frequency or more often if needed. Try to keep humidity at 40% to 60%. If necessary, use a small cool-mist humidifier in the bedroom. This is less dangerous than a hot vaporizer and less expensive than a central humidifier.

From Instructions for Parents, Second Edition, to be published in July 1992, by permission of Sunbelt Medical Publishers, Tallahassee, Florida.

The First Trimester

Usually it is during the first three months (trimester) of your pregnancy that you realize that you are pregnant and come to start your prenatal care. One of the things that will concern you the most is what the APPROXIMATE DATE OF DELIVERY will be. The estimated date is obtained by subtracting three months from the date of your last menstrual period and then adding seven days. This approximation is based on an average 40 weeks of gestation. Remember, this is only an estimate with the average woman delivering within two weeks of the date, either before or after.

During the first trimester your body will undergo a number of changes. Your BREASTS increase in size as the milk-producing tissue increases. You may also notice tenderness in the breasts, tightening of the nipples, and darkening of the nipple area (areola). MORNING SICKNESS does not always occur. If you do experience nausea or vomiting regularly, it is best to contact the practitioner. If only occasionally, try to let the nausea pass. Eat only small frequent meals or things that will be well tolerated such as dry crackers.

Most women experience an increased frequency of URINATION. This is because the enlarged womb puts pressure on the bladder. If there is pain or burning with urination, call the practitioner. The pressure of the womb on the rectum may cause you to develop hemorrhoids. These small outpouchings of enlarged veins can cause you discomfort. If these develop, they should be called to your practitioner's attention. Enlargement of the womb also causes your abdomen to increase in size. Select comfortable maternity clothes that don't compress your belly or restrict circulation in your legs. As the womb enlarges it is better supplied with blood to nourish the fetus. As a result of this increased supply of nutrients, the glands in the mouth of the womb (cervix) produce more mucus which is discharged into the vagina. If there is itchy, odorous, or bloody VAGINAL DISCHARGE, then you should call the practitioner.

Your SKIN, too, will change during pregnancy. Many women will develop reddish-brown blotches on the forehead and cheeks called melasma. These usually fade after pregnancy. Some women will develop a dark line in the middle of the belly that will extend from the pubic area upward toward the top of the abdomen. This line usually fades after the birth of your baby. Some women will develop STRETCH MARKS on the abdomen or breasts. There is probably little that can be done to prevent their development. To some extent they will be of less prominence after delivery.

Many women experience changes in their bowel habits with CONSTIPATION being the frequent problem. To resolve this eat plenty of high bulk foods such as fruits, vegetables, and bran cereals. Prunes and prune juice may also help. If you have INDIGESTION, eat small meals and do not lie down for 30 to 60 minutes after eating.

As your belly gets bigger, you may experience occasional abdominal pain, muscle cramps in the legs, and backache as a result of carrying this extra weight. Try to rest frequently to lessen the strain. To an extent, wearing flat shoes and going barefoot at home will help decrease back discomfort.

When you are pregnant, there are a number of things you should do to ensure your good health and normal fetal development. Get plenty of SLEEP. If you are tired, then you are not getting enough sleep. During pregnancy you need to maintain a high level of CLEANLINESS. During your bath or shower, the nipples and surrounding area should be washed to help toughen the skin. However, go easy on soap, which removes protective oils and dries the skin. You can also toughen the areolar area and nipples by manually pumping your breasts. Sunshine for short periods where you won't get arrested for indecent exposure will also help toughen the skin. Vaginal hygiene is always of concern. Simple washing of the external genitals should be sufficient. It is not necessary to douche, spray, or disinfect the vagina which is, after all, not supposed to be sterile, and these practices may be harmful during pregnancy.

It is very important to follow a well balanced DIET. It is not necessary to restrict your weight increase unless you were overweight prior to becoming pregnant. You can expect to gain _____ lbs/kg. It is important to eat a moderate but sufficient amount of nutritious calories, approximately 2500 a day. Try to limit starches, pastries, candies, and other sweets which are not healthful. Each day you should have several servings of protein such as meat and eggs (or other protein sources), cheese, milk or milk products. The latter also supply calcium for development of the fetus. Vitamins, too, are important. If you eat a well balanced diet, including raw fruit and vegetables, you are probably getting most of the recommended vitamins with the exception of folic acid and getting most of the recommended minerals with the exception of iron. Consequently, vitamin and mineral supplements are recommended.

There are a number of things that should not be done during pregnancy. Cigarette SMOKING is absolutely forbidden. Smoking during pregnancy decreases the birth weight of the child and increases the chance of premature birth. Smokers frequently have miscarriages. ALCOHOL should be avoided. No drugs. NO MEDICATIONS should be taken without being approved by the doctor. This includes not taking medicines available without a prescription such as aspirin, laxatives, cold medicines.

There are a number of other areas that concern expectant parents with regard to SEXUAL RELATIONS. You should simply follow your desires. During the last four weeks, you may have difficulty in the usual positions for relations, and other positions may have to be tried. Do not engage in sexual relations once labor has begun or membranes have ruptured.

EXERCISES to which you are accustomed can be continued. Now is not the time to take up running obstacle courses or the marathon--which can jeopardize your pregnancy. Other exercises will be recommended during your pregnancy. Never push yourself to the point of exhaustion or of experiencing pain.

Most women can continue to WORK throughout their pregnancy. A job with several physical or emotional demands could be detrimental. If you have questions about your job, these should be discussed, but otherwise continue as long as you want to and are able--even until you go into labor. It's hell sitting at home waiting for a baby to come when you are not at all used to that role.

During the first trimester you will be giving a complete physical. You will also be tested for anemia. A number of other tests on your blood will be performed. A number of vaginal tests will be performed, including a Pap smear. Depending on your age or past of family history, genetic testing may be recommended. You will be seen regularly to monitor your health and the development of your baby. You will be examined at regular intervals, particularly examining your belly to follow the growth of your womb and development of the fetus. Periodic fetal assessment may be performed. Blood pressure, urine, and other tests will be done periodically to see that complications are not developing.

Again, your practitioner/doctor should be contacted if you have bloody or odorous vaginal discharge, burning when urinating, persistent headache, severe nausea and vomiting, swelling of the hands, feet, or face, are will with a fever, or have abdominal pain not relieved by a bowel movement.

Additional Resources

Nursing Your Baby by Karen Pryor. This is an easy to read book that will help you prepare for the nursing experience. Husbands should read this also. As an alternative, consider reading The Womanly Art of Breast Feeding from La Leche League, 1-800-423-0102.

Consider the use of an exercise video, The American College of Obstetricians and Gynecologists Pregnancy Exercise Program. They also published a new book, Planning for Pregnancy and Beyond. Order from 1-800-543-6016.

Pregnancy and Childbirth by Sheila Kitzinger has a new updated version and is an excellent book to prepare a woman for the changes of pregnancy and for a natural childbirth experience.

From Instructions for Parents, Second Edition, to be published in July 1992, by permission of Sunbelt Medical Publishers, Tallahassee, Florida.

Acne

What Is It?
Acne is a usually self-limiting inflammatory disease of the oil-producing glands and follicles in the skin.

What Are the Symptoms?
Acne is characterized by the occlusion of these glands. The material which plugs the pores is a mixture of oil and skin protein called a whitehead. Exposure of this mixture to air causes it to darken, hence the term blackhead (comedones). Pimples are the result of inflammation of the surrounding skin. These acne lesions may become infected or form cysts.

How Long Does It Last?
It is impossible to predict how long you/your child will have acne. Acne rarely carries over from adolescence to adulthood.

What Are the Complications?
Infected or cystic lesions may cause permanent scars.

How Common Is It?
More than three fourths of all preadolescents or adolescents have acne. Fewer than 15% of these have it severely.

How Is It Acquired?
Acne occurs in those who have inherited a tendency for developing acne. It begins at the time that a child's body is undergoing hormonal changes associated with maturation.

What Can the Family Do?
You/your child is concerned about his/her appearance and therefore should read this material and try to assume the responsibility for treatment. Parents should aid in providing for medical visits and in paying for medicines.

A number of measures are helpful in treating acne. Eliminating certain foods (except those which seem to make your acne worse) has no value. Though keeping the skin clean is important, it can be overdone. Abrasive soaps (those which contain pumice or granules) and astringents (alcohol based preparations for removing oil) can make things worse by irritating the oil producing glands. It is best to wash gently with a mild soap several times a day. Squeezing pimples and blackheads can cause skin damage. Sunlight (particularly the ultraviolet component) is helpful, but care must be taken to prevent burning and eye damage.

What Has the Doctor Done?
Acne therapy must be individualized. Additionally, therapy may need to be changed from time to time. Carefully following the instructions given usually results in considerable improvement. You may not need additional costly ineffective over-the-counter preparations.

When To Call the Doctor Again
The practitioner will want to examine your child at regular intervals to monitor therapy and adjust medications and in certain instances monitor for adverse effects of medications.

From Instructions for Parents, Second Edition, to be published in July 1992, by permission of Sunbelt Medical Publishers, Tallahassee, Florida.

Dry Skin

Dry skin contributes to the discomfort you or your child experience in a number of conditions. People with dry skin have a problem losing water through the skin either all over or in those areas that itch or have a rash. There are quite a number of things that can be done to make you or your child more comfortable.

1. Help to keep the skin moist by taking warm soaking baths (this allows the skin to absorb water). Fifteen to 20 minutes once or twice daily should be sufficient. If the water is too hot it will promote itching. Avoid bubble baths. Use a therapeutic bath oil in the water _____ or add oilated colloidal oatmeal _____ which has the added advantage of helping soothe itching.

2. During bathing try to avoid use of soaps altogether. But, if this is not possible use a mild soap _____ or a non-alkaline skin cleanser _____.
Be careful too, about the choice of shampoos which may add considerable soap to the water and defeat the purpose of these other bathing measures.

3. After bathing lightly pat the skin dry. While still damp apply an appropriate level of an agent to seal in the moisture. The mildest is to use a vegetable or bath oil. Thicker agents are better sealants but have the disadvantage being greasy.
Consider moisturizers _____
                              and/or
consider emollients _____.

4. Avoid scratchy irritating clothes and bedding. Woolens may be the most offending. But consider changing to milder laundry detergents and using an extra rinse cycle. Be careful if you or your child is sensitive to fabric softeners, then add this to the first rinse (never to the drier). Never wear new clothes or use new bedding that has not been previously and thoroughly washed.

5. Keep fingernails short and avoid/discourage scratching.

6. Avoid all "itch" creams, lotions and gels unless recommended by the nurse practitioner or the physician.

7. In dry climates, dry seasons, or when the heat is on at home, consider running a cool mist humidifier. This may be particularly valuable in the bedroom. These are safer than vaporizers as no one gets burnt if one is knocked over.

8. If stress is a contributing factor then discuss relaxation techniques.

9. If this a new problem, re-examine your home and work/school environment, hobbies and habits for possible irritants and contributing factors.

Poison Ivy, Poison Oak, and Poison Sumac

What Is It?
Poison ivy, poison oak, or poison sumac is a rash on exposed parts of the body that come in contact with any part of these plants. It usually occurs in the spring and summer when children are outdoors but can occur any time of the year. The rash occurs only in those people sensitive to an oily substance produced by members of the Rhus plant family, renamed the Toxicodendron family. This sensitivity is a reaction by you/your child's body to previous exposure to this substance. The skin must usually be in contact with the oil for several hours to cause a reaction. The rash can begin up to several days after this contact.

What Are the Symptoms?
The rash usually appears as clusters of small blisters or pimples on reddened skin. The blisters may leak a fluid which can dry and crust. You/your child may be suffering intense itching and scratch constantly.

How Long Does It Last?
Poison ivy, poison oak, or poison sumac rashes are usually present for several weeks.

What Are the Complications?
The areas involved can become infected with bacteria and leak pus.

How Common Is It?
These rashes are very common. Children who are sensitive may have it often and severely.

How Is It Acquired?
You/your child developed this rash because of contact with the Rhus oil. This oil may be on any part of these plants and on mango skin or in mango sap. The oil, unless removed from the skin, can be spread to other areas on skin or even to other individuals. However, fluids from the blisters will not cause spread of the rash. Pets, clothing, or other outdoor equipment can have the oil on their hair or surfaces and consequently serve as a source of the rash. The smoke from burning trash (which has Rhus plants or parts) contains oil and can cause the skin reaction.

What Can the Family Do?
Several measures may be taken to relieve your child's itching discomfort. Moist, cold compresses can be applied to these affected areas to obtain relief. Cool baths xor showers may also be temporarily helpful. Some physicians advocate a good hot shower or bath at bedtime, which temporarily makes the itching worse but, in doing so, depletes you/your child's reaction. This may help provide a good night's sleep. Many people obtain relief with calamine lotion (which can occasionally cause a skin reaction of its own, making things worse).

Skin damage and spread of infection may be lessened by keeping you/your child's fingernails short.

Most importantly, teach yourself and your older children to recognize the plants of the Rhus family. Teach them, too, to avoid these plants or places where they might grow. If you/your child is going camping or participating in other situations in which he/she might contact these plants, long pants and shirts will decrease the possibility of skin contact. These clothes should be removed and washed as soon thereafter as possible.

The family should take **measures to prevent the spread of the oil**. Vigorous washing with soap and water of the body is of prime importance to remove all of the oily substance. The quicker the oil is washed away, the less will be absorbed, decreasing the amount and severity of the rash. Removing the oil will also prevent the spread of rash. These measures are particularly important if you/your child come in contact again with these plants or the oil. Removal of the oil will not prevent occurrence of the rash in the areas already having sufficient contact. New rash can appear more than a week after initial contact. All clothing should be washed.

What Has the Doctor Done?
Your practitioner/doctor may have prescribed medicine to apply to the areas involved or a medicine to be taken by mouth to relieve the itching. Severe cases may require more individualized therapy.

When To Call the Doctor Again
The physician should be called if you/your child's rash is becoming infected or if the symptoms are worsening. If possible, this should be done during regular office hours.

From Instructions for Parents, Second Edition, to be published in July 1992, by permission of Sunbelt Medical Publishers, Tallahassee, Florida.

Mini-Mental Status Examination

	Maximum score	Patient's score
Orientation		
What is the year, season, date, day and month?	5	_____
Where are we? (state, county, town, hospital and floor)	5	_____
Registration		
Name three objects (allow the patient one second to say each). Ask the patient to say all three after you have said them. Then repeat the names of the three objects until the patient learns all three. Count the number of trials and record: _____	3	_____
Attention and calculation		
Serial 7's (1 point for each correct answer). Stop after five answers. Or, spell "world" backwards.	5	_____
Recall		
Ask the patient to name the three objects mentioned previously. (Score 1 point for each correct answer.)	3	_____
Language		
Name a pencil and a watch.	2	_____
Repeat the following: "No ifs, ands or buts."	1	_____
Follow a three-stage command: "Take a paper in your right hand, fold it in half and put it on the floor."	3	_____
Read and obey the following: "Close your eyes."	1	_____
Write a sentence.	1	_____
Copy design.	1	_____
Total possible score:	30	

Check one: Alert _____ Drowsy _____ Stuporous _____ Comatose _____

Instructions for administering the mini-mental status examination

Orientation
Ask for the date. Then ask specifically for the parts omitted (e.g., "Can you also tell me what season it is?"). Score 1 point for each correct answer. Ask in turn "Can you tell me the name of this hospital?" (town, county, etc.). Score 1 point for each correct answer.

Registration
Ask the patient if you may test his memory. Then say the names of three unrelated objects, clearly and slowly, about one second for each. After you have said all three, ask the patient to repeat the names. This first repetition determines the score (0-3), but keep saying them until the patient can repeat all three, up to six trials. If the patient does not eventually learn all three, recall cannot be meaningfully tested.

Attention and calculation
Ask the patient to begin with 100 and count backwards by seven. Stop after five subtractions (93, 86, 79, 72, 65). Score the total number of correct answers. If the patient cannot or will not perform this task, ask him to spell the word "world" backwards. The score is the number of letters in correct order (e.g., dlrow = 5, dlorw = 3).

Recall
Ask the patient if he can recall the three words you previously asked him to remember. Score 0-3.

Language
Naming: Show the patient a wrist watch and ask him what it is. Repeat for a pencil. Score 0-2.
Repetition: Ask the patient to repeat the sentence after you. Allow only one trial. Score 0 or 1.
Three-stage command: Give the patient a piece of plain blank paper and repeat the command. Score 1 point for each part correctly executed.
Reading: On a blank piece of paper, print the sentence "Close your eyes," in letters large enough for the patient to see clearly. Ask the patient to read it and do what it says. Score 1 point only if the patient actually closes his eyes.
Writing: Give the patient a blank piece of paper and ask him to write a sentence for you. Do not dictate a sentence; it must be written spontaneously. It must contain a subject and verb, and it must be sensible. Correct grammar and punctuation are not necessary.
Copying: On a clean piece of paper, draw intersecting pentagons, each side about 1 in, and ask the patient to copy it exactly as it is.

Sensorium
Estimate the patient's level of sensorium along a continuum, from alert on the left to comatose on the right.

Reprinted with permission from Journal of Psychiatric Research, vol. 12, M. F. Folstein, "Mini-Mental Status Exam," 1975, Pergamon Press, Inc.

INDEX

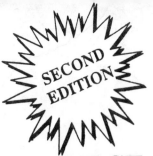

SAVE TIME!
BUY
NURSE PRACTITIONER PROTOCOLS

By Matthew M. Cohen, M.D., FAFP
and Anni Lanigan, ARNP, FNP-C

SUNBELT MEDICAL PUBLISHERS

Save yourself and your physician-employer time!

Three-ring Binder Edition:
Single copy . . . .$85.00 each
3-10 copies . . . .$70.00 each
11-50 copies . . . .$55.00 each

Soft Cover Edition:
Single copy . . . .$50.00 each
3-10 copies . . . .$41.50 each
11-50 copies . . . .$35.00 each

Prices Subject to Change Without Notice

Sunbelt Medical Publishers:
P. O. Box 13512 Dept. PP
Tallahassee, Florida 32317-3512

Shipping and Handling:
1 copy . . . .$10.00 each
2-5 copies . . . .$ 5.00 each
5 or more copies . . . .$ 3.50 each
Florida residents add 7% sales tax.

DESCRIPTION	QUANTITY	PRICE	TOTAL

SUNBELT MEDICAL PUBLISHERS

Make your check payable to:
Sunbelt Medical Publishers:
P. O. Box 13512 Dept. PP
Tallahassee, Florida 32317-3512

7% SALES TAX _____
SHIPPING & HANDLING _____
TOTAL ENCLOSED _____

Allow 6-8 weeks for delivery.

Ship to: Name _____

Street Address _____

City _____ State _____ Zip _____

DESCRIPTION	QUANTITY	PRICE	TOTAL

SUNBELT MEDICAL PUBLISHERS

Make your check payable to:
Sunbelt Medical Publishers:
P. O. Box 13512 Dept. PP
Tallahassee, Florida 32317-3512

7% SALES TAX _____
SHIPPING & HANDLING _____
TOTAL ENCLOSED _____

Allow 6-8 weeks for delivery.

Ship to: Name _____

Street Address _____

City _____ State _____ Zip _____